Mental Health in Children & Adolescents

A Guide for Teachers

Sarah Buckley MB, MRCPsych

Blánaid Gavin MB, MRCPsych

Fiona McNicholas MD, FRCPsych

First published 2009

ISBN 978-0-9551241-8-1

British Library Cataloguing in Publication Data.
A catalogue record for this publication is available from the British Library

Printed in Ireland by Colorman, Dublin.

Published by Mulberry Publications, 24 Melrose Avenue, Drogheda, Ireland.

Contents

Preface

'There is no health without mental health'.

Mental illness has been described as the 'chronic disease of the young' as it is more common than physical illness in young people. Indeed 75% of all adult mental health difficulties begin before twenty-four years of age. Like so many medical illnesses, the quicker a person receives effective treatment the greater the likelihood of successful response to that treatment. Furthermore, the earlier effective intervention is instigated the greater the impact on illness outcome.

However, mental health difficulties in children and teenagers are often unrecognised. Consequently, young people commonly go without treatment which is known to be effective and this occurs at a crucial developmental stage when they should be laying the foundations for their personal, academic and economic advancement. When seen in a developmental context, the negative impact of untreated mental health difficulties is readily apparent: a child's developmental trajectory may be significantly derailed due to an inability to perform to his or her social and academic potential.

The Irish government's mental health policy, *A Vision for Change* (2006), recognises the morbidity associated with youth mental health problems and advocates for a comprehensive mental health service across the entire community. The role that schools and teachers can play in promoting positive mental health in children should not be underestimated. Creating a school ethos which promotes and builds strengths amongst students whatever their academic profile, can turn risk into resilience and significantly reduce the prevalence and impact of mental health disorders. It is hoped that this book on mental health in young people will be a useful resource to you as you continue to work to enrich the lives of the children that come your way.

Acknowledgements

The authors would like to thank the St. John of God Research Grants Committee which provided the funding for this book. We would also like to thank Mr. Paddy O'Dwyer, Director, National Educational Psychological Service, for commenting on an earlier draft of this book and providing us with very useful feedback. We would particularly like to thank the teachers who participated in our Focus Groups on CAMHs and Schools. The insights provided by the teachers who participated was instrumental in prompting us to write this book. Finally, we would like to extend our gratitude to Ms. Marie McCourt, Lucena Foundation for all her kind help with this project.

1 Introduction

What is Mental Illness?

Many people have emotional difficulties from time to time such as brief periods of feeling sad, anxious, inadequate or stressed. However, the experience of severe symptoms lasting for a substantial period of time coupled with significant impairment in personal, social and educational or occupational aspects of life are what differentiates minor mental health difficulties from mental illness.

Mental illness is therefore described as: the experience of severe and distressing psychological symptoms to the extent that normal functioning is seriously impaired and help (medication, psychotherapy or lifestyle change) is needed to facilitate recovery.

All mental illnesses are classified in a book called the DSM IV (Diagnostic Statistic Manual version IV, American Psychiatric Association), or an equivalent book, International Classification of Diseases (ICD 10, World Health Organisation). These books are regularly updated by field research. Throughout this book we will refer specifically to the criteria required by DSM IV to make a diagnosis.

Prevalence of Mental Illness

Mental illness is much more common than physical illness in young people. Therefore mental illness has been described as the 'chronic disease of the

1

young'(McGorry, 2009). 75% of all mental health difficulties have begun before twenty-four years of age.

Why focus on Mental Illness in Children and Adolescents?

There are a number of compelling reasons why it is important to recognise and treat mental health difficulties in children and teenagers, as regrettably most are unrecognised and untreated. This leads to significant associated morbidity and mortality. Furthermore mental health difficulties are the leading cause of lifelong disability with a very high risk of persistence into adulthood when untreated. The negative impact of mental health difficulties across multiple domains of a young person's life is very powerful particularly on education, physical health and families. Detecting early signs of difficulty and providing effective treatment can potentially prevent the substantial secondary negative consequences of childhood mental illness.

How Common is Mental Illness in Young People?

The numbers of young people struggling with mental health difficulties without help is a major public health concern. The causes for the apparent increase in some psychiatric illnesses are unclear but are thought to be mainly sociological.

- ➤ 1 in 5 young people have psychological problems;
- ➤ 1 in 10 young people have mental illness with some impairment (when some form of psychological help is usually required);
- ➤ 1 in 20 young people have a major psychiatric disorder;
- ➤ 1 in 200 young people require in-patient admission to a psychiatric unit.

The following groups of children are at higher risk of mental health difficulties:

- ➤ Children who are/were victims of abuse;
- ➤ Children whose parents have mental illness;
- ➤ Children with physical illness;
- ➤ Children with learning disability;
- ➤ Children from the Travelling Community.

A study to establish the rates of psychiatric illness in school-going teenagers in Dublin was recently carried out (Lynch and Fitzpatrick et al, 2007). This study was carried out on over seven hundred 12-15 year olds attending secondary school. The following rates of psychiatric disorder were detected:

Table 1.1

Any Psychiatric disorder	15.6%
Depression	4.5%
Suicidal Ideation	1.9%
Anxiety	3.7%
ADHD	3.7%
Conduct Disorder	2.4%
Tics	1.1%
Eating Disorder	0.2%

It is worth noting that many psychiatric illnesses have their peak incidents later in adolescence so these figures are likely to be an underestimate of the prevalence rates of mental health difficulties in students in the senior cycle of secondary school. Furthermore children with the most severe mental health difficulties are much more likely to be absent from school and therefore not included in prevalence studies such as these.

Mental Health Promotion

Schools have an important role in the recognition of mental health problems in children and in the provision of an environment that fosters mental well-being. Research has shown that mental health promotion and prevention programmes have significant benefits for children and adolescents. Children with emotional, behavioural or social difficulties may need extra support to learn and benefit from the school environment. If all children are to reach their full potential the education system must be a system that can be flexible and accommodate their needs.

Mental health promotion aims to facilitate mental well-being and to address the needs of those at risk of or experiencing mental health problems. The goal of mental health promotion is the enhancement of potential and to build on psychological strengths and resilience. To overcome the problems of stigma and denial it is important that mental health is promoted as "everyone's business".

Mentally healthy children can achieve the following:

➢ Initiate, develop, and sustain mutually satisfying personal relationships;
➢ Use and enjoy solitude;
➢ Become aware of others and empathise with them;
➢ Play and learn;
➢ Develop a sense of right and wrong;
➢ Resolve problems and set backs and learn from them.

A Vision for Change (2006) which is now government policy is a comprehensive model of mental health service provision for Ireland. It recommends that positive mental health is built across the entire community. It also recommends that SPHE (Social, Personal and Health Education Curriculum) extends to secondary school. SPHE helps children learn skills to be competent to learn about themselves and others and to make informed decisions about their health, personal and social life. It enables children to develop a framework for responsible decision making and provides opportunities for reflection and discussion.

Students who have participated in mental health programmes report an increased ability to cope with problems and emotions and improved interpersonal relations. These programmes have also been shown to enhance learning achievements and overall educational attainments. With the increasing emphasis on educational achievement and performance indicators, it is important that care is taken to ensure that the school strives to support emotional development. When children are attending mental health services they may have ongoing difficulties which a positive school environment can significantly ameliorate.

Many children with mental health difficulties present challenging behaviour in the classroom. Teachers should have strategies in place to encourage positive behaviour and to identify children with behaviour difficulties secondary to mental health problems. Teachers can provide a forum for children to 'open up' about such problems by facilitating discussions during SPHE. It can also be helpful to use a 'worry box' or to ask children to draw their worries as a class exercise.

School ethos has been described as the "curricular and organisational features of the school which communicate certain values to the school community and thereby help promote the development of fundamental values in children" (Atkinson & Hornby, 2002). It requires commitment, leadership, equal opportunities, valuing diversity and clear policies on behavioural expectations. It is important to promote a collaborative rather than a competitive approach and encourage children to work together rather than against each other.

It is important that children develop a sense of community in school. Just as academic success is rewarded and praised, student behaviour which is inclusive and promotes cooperation should be commended. When a school is functioning well, if a child becomes distressed or is under pressure other children are more likely to help their classmate and inform a teacher.

If children learn through experience that they are an important part of the school and can make contributions which are valued they will be motivated to engage positively in the school community. Simple steps such as displaying children's work will encourage involvement and appreciation of the school ethos. Children should be involved in the development of school guidelines such as bullying policies or a 'Buddy System'.

Children with mental health problems may have many challenges in order to succeed in school. They may miss school and fall behind in their academic work and often require extra assistance from the teacher when they return. They may be too worried or upset to concentrate and may not be able to learn properly. They may become isolated and this may further compound such worries and feelings. It is important that other children are supportive of pupils who may be struggling in class and include them in peer activities.

A child is more likely to make progress with difficulties where there is clear consistent communication between school and home as this helps to ensure that the child is getting the same message from authority figures in both settings. Although it can be time-consuming to establish close links with parents, it will ultimately help the teacher understand the context in which a child is living. Close links between parents and school facilitate sharing of useful information such as strategies which parents use to calm the child. It is particularly helpful if both parents and teachers have an agreed plan, focusing on areas in which the child is experiencing difficulties. Parents are more likely to 'buy into' plans which include their views and suggestions. If a child is on medication, it is very important for teachers to inform parents of any changes in a child's behaviour or academic progress.

To be available to learn new skills, children need to feel safe physically and emotionally . School rules regarding acceptable behaviour and bullying must be explicit. Every school should have a strong anti-bullying ethos and a clear protocol to deal with bullying should it happen.

Teachers should promote non-violent resolution of conflicts among the children. Any incident must be effectively dealt with as soon as possible. If teachers identify any particular incidents of concern, these should be investigated; it is important to be particularly vigilant during break-time when incidents of bullying are more likely to occur.

The 'Friends' programme which is a school based universal bullying prevention programme is very useful. It consists of ten sessions which the teachers deliver in school, followed by two booster sessions. The programme promotes important self-development concepts such as self-esteem, problem-solving, psychological resilience, self-expression and building positive relationships with peers and adults.

It is also important that teachers feel safe in the school. There have been reports of teachers being bullied by pupils, pupils' parents and colleagues. Clear guidelines must be explained to all children and their parents on entry into school and there should be a clear plan of action to follow if a complaint of bullying is made.

Access to a school counsellor can help children and is potentially less stigmatising than attending a mental health service. This can be of great support to a child who becomes distressed in class and may need a short break from the classroom. This form of supportive and relatively low-key intervention may be sufficient to calm the child and make the school day tolerable. This enables a child to stay for a longer school day in a very supportive environment.

Teachers need ongoing support and training to help to develop an understanding of what mental health problems are and how to support children with these difficulties in school. Often it is useful to have some training as part of an in-service day or summer training programme. Knowledge of and attitudes towards Mental Health and behaviour affect both teachers and pupils attending the school. Sometimes senior teachers may be available for peer support and can share ideas they have found useful and this can be of great benefit for all the group.

Special Education Support Service

The SESS was established in September 2003. The service co-ordinates, develops and delivers a range of professional development initiatives and support structures for school personnel working with students with special educational needs in a variety of educational settings. These settings include mainstream primary and post-primary schools, special schools and special classes attached to mainstream schools.

Resources Available for Children with Special Education Needs

General Allocation of Resources. Department of Education and Science, circular 02/05. Categories of Low-Incidence Special Educational Needs. (Please note that this allocation is due to be revised and is correct at the time of writing).This section sets out the various categories of low incidence disabilities and the level of resource teaching support available to schools in respect of each category.

The general allocation model provides additional teaching resources to assist schools in making appropriate provision for:

- pupils who are eligible for learning-support teaching;
- pupils with learning difficulties;
- pupils who have special educational needs arising from high incidence disabilities (borderline mild general learning disability, mild general learning disability and specific learning disability).

Each school individually decides how the resources for high incidence support should be used and how these resources are divided amongst the students who need this support.

Parents of children with Specific Speech and Language Disorders may apply to the Special Educational Needs Organiser (SENO) to establish a special class with at least five eligible pupils in it.

Table 1.2

Low Incidence Disabilities	Hours of resource teaching support available to school per week
Physical Disability	3
Hearing Impairment	4
Visual Impairment	3.5
Emotional Disturbance	3.5
Severe Emotional Disturbance	5
Moderate General Learning Disability	3.5
Severe / Profound General Learning Disability	5
Autism / Autistic Spectrum Disorders	5
Specific Speech and Language Disorder	4
Assessed syndrome in conjunction with one of the above low incidence disabilities	3 to 5, taking into account the pupil's special educational needs including level of general learning disability
Multiple Disabilities	5

Learning/Intellectual Disability and Risk of Mental Illness

Many children may have specific learning disabilities (reading, writing or maths) but may have a normal IQ and perform very well in other areas. It is always important to make sure that all children have their vision and hearing checked as this can have a significant impact on a child's ability to learn.

Children are considered to have a general learning disability or intellectual disability if they have an IQ of less than 70 points on cognitive assessment. Children with an IQ of 55 - 70 are in the mild range of learning disability and many manage in mainstream schools but often need additional learning support. Children with lower IQs may require special schools for children with moderate to severe learning disability.

Having a general learning disability impacts on a child's development and often includes difficulties with attention, difficulty understanding instruction, delayed speech and language skills and behaviour that is immature for his or her age. Many children have significant difference between their oral and written performance and it is very important that this is fully assessed to maximise learning potential for the child.

Statistically, children with a general learning disability have a higher rate of mental health problems which often contribute to difficulties in school. The prevalence of mental health problems is considered to be two and a half to four times higher in children with an intellectual disability than in children with normal intelligence. Mental health problems are often overlooked due to the issue of 'diagnostic overshadowing' whereby there is a tendency to overlook psychological and emotional problems in children with an intellectual disability.

It is very important where a child has a mental health problem as well as a learning disability that this is detected as soon as possible so that appropriate intervention is made available.

Promoting Well-being

Resilience

The majority of children and adolescents manage to cope successfully with a variety of challenging situations in their lives. There has been increased recognition of this in the recent psychological literature leading to a drive to define the attributes that allow young people overcome adverse life circumstances. The concept of resilience has been described by Krovetz, a former high-school principal, as 'the belief in the ability of every person to overcome adversity if important protective factors are present in a person's life'. While the concept of resilience has been increasingly recognized in psychology, its potential role in the field of education has been less extensively explored with some notable exceptions. Krowetz has described 'resilient school communities' which attempt to foster resilience both in the students and teachers. The International Resilience Project collected data from 30 countries and defined resilience as 'a universal capacity which allows a person, group or community to prevent, minimise or overcome the damaging effects of adversity'. All participating countries presented a similar range of factors which were associated with resilience indicating that these factors crossed cultural boundaries. The authors of the Resilience Project Report defined resilient children as 'better equipped to resist stress and adversity, cope with change and uncertainty and to recover faster and more completely from traumatic events or episodes'.

Resilience is a dynamic rather than a static attribute and as such can emerge at different times in a young person's life. The four attributes that have been most consistently associated with resilience are:

> ## 1. Social Competence
> This includes the ability to seek help from peers in addition to adults as well as the ability to elicit positive responses from others.

> ## 2. Problem-solving skills
> This describes a child who has the ability to work out how to deal with problems as they arise, has confidence in general and specifically an ability to problem-solve.

> ## 3. Autonomy
> This is defined as an ability to think and act independently while having a clear sense of personal identity.

> ## 4. Sense of Purpose
> This is defined as having meaningful goals and belief in the future.

It is thought that these attributes are most likely to lead to resilience in an environment which is caring and provides positive expectations and facilitates participation which is viewed as meaningful by the young person.

Table 1.3 Resilience Factors

The Child	The Family	The Environment
Temperament (Good-natured) Feelings of empathy, internal locus of control Humour, Attractiveness	Caring Parents who are supportive	Supportive extended family
Gender: Female prior to and male during adolescence	Good parent-child relationships	Experience of success in school
Age (younger age)	Good Parental Relationship	Friendship
Cognitive Ability (Higher IQ)	Valued role within family	Valued role within community
Good Social skills	Close relationship with one parent	Mentor who provides support
Personal awareness		Member of religious community

Self–Esteem

Self-esteem is extremely important in order for children to fulfil their potential. Self-esteem is defined as the individual's appraisal of self. Self-image and ideal-self are integral components of self-esteem. Self-esteem reflects the difference between children's perception of how they are (self-image) and how they ideally would like to be (ideal-self).

Self-esteem develops in the context of children's appraisal of their life experiences. For example, one child may have an awareness of poor academic skills which may be balanced by a positive sense of social competence. Whereas another child might struggle in all domains and again be very aware of this.

Childrens's self-esteem is also influenced by the value placed on their abilities by those close to them. For example, one child may struggle with reading but have a parent who ensures that the child is supported appropriately and self-esteem may be unaffected. Another child may be subjected to harsh criticism from parents in the same situation which will have a negative impact on self-esteem.

Both mental health and learning have foundations in self-esteem and therefore it is an important area to focus on in schools (Rutter et al, 1998). Often achievement in schools is measured in terms of academic performance. If a child continues to do badly in this area, the effect on confidence and self-esteem can be detrimental.

Problem–solving skills

The development of coping skills and problem-solving ability is an essential part of growing up. All young people encounter a range of challenges to a greater or lesser extent during their school-going years. The approach the young person takes to the problem whether big or small is an essential learning experience and provides a template for how the individual deals with potentially greater challenges in later life. Young people can be helped to enhance their problem-solving skills.

Problem solving is a sequence. Firstly, a person must realise that a problem exists. Next it is necessary to put the problem in words and describe the feelings that the problem evokes. Alternative solutions should then be generated and the steps required to achieve these must be worked out. Finally the child needs to be able to anticipate consequences and make appropriate decisions. It is possible to generate imaginary scenarios in the class to facilitate successful problem-solving. Pupils can be encouraged to 'brainstorm' solutions following the RIBEYE steps outlined below.

RIBEYE

* **R**ecognize that there is a problem
* **I**dentify what the problem is
* **B**rainstorm about the solution
* **E**valuate the solution
* **Y**es - to one solution
* **E**ncourage and praise the child for a job well done

Emotional Intelligence

Many young people have significant deficits in their ability to identify and to regulate emotions. As a result, they have a reduced ability to use emotions to guide thought processes and to prioritise thinking. They may also find it difficult to identify and understand emotions in others.

Accurate detection, labelling and understanding of emotional states is very important to mental well-being. It is crucial that children acquire the competence to recognize and manage emotions, develop concern for others, establish positive relationships, make responsible decisions and handle challenging situations effectively. This will support children in their personal, social, family and academic life.

Emotions are important for communication. Well developed emotional skills can protect against adversity and facilitate coping when challenges arise. Emotions cannot be separated from cognitive and social skills and are linked to attention, memory, learning, decision-making, and quality relationships. Emotions have an adaptive value as pleasant emotions lead to creativity and can improve relationships. Negative emotions may also have adaptive value, for example when channelling anger in a constructive way.

Emotional literacy helps students to recognize and label their emotions and those of others, to understand the causes of their emotions, to express and communicate their feelings effectively and to regulate their emotions to enhance relationships and academic functioning. Emotional literacy determines how well we understand and express ourselves, and understand and relate to others.

Socially, emotional literacy helps students to develop self-awareness, empathy, communication skills, problem-solving skills and healthy relationships. Academically, emotional literacy enhances vocabulary, reading comprehension, creativity and critical thinking.

Child and Adolescent Mental Health Services (CAMHS)

What problems do Child and Adolescent Mental Health Services deal with?

Child and Adolescent Mental Health Services deal with a broad range of mental health difficulties including all of those covered in this book. Emotional and behavioural problems in young people are common. The function of CAMHS is to help young people and their families by diagnosing their difficulty, providing them with information about it, and planning treatment that will improve their psychological well-being.

It is important to remember that some mental health problems which are typically associated with adulthood, such as Schizophrenia, Eating Disorders and Bipolar Affective Disorder may also begin in childhood and consequently may be treated by CAMHS.

When is a child seen by CAMHS?

A child is seen when concerns have been raised regarding a child's psychological well-being. In some CAMHS clinics the child must be referred by a medical doctor (for example: GP, Area Medical Officer or Paediatrician) to be put on the clinic waiting list. If this is the case, the concerned person, for example, the Teacher, Social Worker or National Educational Psychologist should recommend to the parent that the child be brought to a GP so a decision can be reached as to the need for referral to a CAMHS clinic.

In clinics that do not require medical referral, any concerned professional, or the parent themselves, can refer the child. The decision as to which particular CAMHS clinic the child is referred is based on the address at which the child resides, as mental health services operate by catchment area. Once the referral is received, the child is put on the clinic waiting list for assessment. Urgent cases are prioritised and seen very quickly but others may be some time on a routine waiting list for assessment. Urgent cases include children who are suicidal or psychotic.

Where are Child and Adolescent Mental Health Services based?

In Ireland the vast majority of CAMHS teams operate through outpatient clinics, either in stand alone buildings or linked with a hospital or other clinical services. However, there are also a small number of day-patient and inpatient facilities. Young people who require more in-depth assessment or require greater therapeutic input than that which is available through an outpatient department may be referred to these units. In a day-hospital, for example, the child may attend a number of times per week for a number of hours. Inpatient psychiatric beds are extremely limited and are generally reserved for children with severe symptoms which cannot be managed in either out-patient or day-patient setting. It is thought that only 0.5-1% of the child population require an in-patient admission.

What does an initial assessment consist of?

Generally both parents and child are seen at the first assessment. It is important to get a comprehensive picture of the child's difficulties and to consider apparent problems in a child, which may be better understood in the context of problems in either parent or in the context of environmental factors. The assessment will be carried out by one or more members of the multidisciplinary team and may last up to two hours.

Over the course of the assessment, a range of issues is explored including the child's current difficulties, any past psychological problems and any early developmental difficulties. The child's early years are discussed. The child's experience in school, both from an educational and social perspective, is considered. The family history including parents, siblings and extended family is explored both in terms of the history of psychological difficulties in the family and the relationships and communication within the family. The information that is gathered in the initial session allows the development of a 'differential diagnosis' which is a list of potential explanations for the child's current difficulties. The purpose of the subsequent assessments is to accurately establish the diagnosis which will inform the intervention provided.

What are the predictors of poor response to treatment?

The type and severity of symptoms is the best indicator of prognosis. However, a variety of additional factors can result in poorer response to treatment. Predictors of response to treatment are very general and may not apply in any one specific case.

The following are predictors of poorer treatment response:

> ➢ Children with socio-economic disadvantage;
> ➢ Poor educational background of parents;
> ➢ Parental discord;
> ➢ Single parent status;
> ➢ Parental psychiatric disturbance;
> ➢ Significantly disturbed relationship between parent and child;
> ➢ Poor relationship between child and therapist.

Why are there different professionals on CAMHS teams?

There are different professionals working together on Child and Adolescent Mental Health teams to enable a comprehensive assessment and treatment of the difficulties the child presents with. Each different discipline brings a different skill to the team. The mix of disciplines involved in the assessment and treatment of the child will depend on the nature of the child's difficulties. This is known to be the best way to help children with mental health difficulties.

Who are the members of the multidisciplinary team?

> ➢ The multidisciplinary team may include:
>
> **Child Psychiatrist**: Child Psychiatrists are medically qualified doctors who have specialised in working in mental health with young people. Their expertise lies in understanding and working with children who have mental health difficulties. Child Psychiatrists can diagnose specific mental illnesses and advise on treatment options. They also have training in pharmacology and are able to prescribe medication when appropriate.
>
> ➢ **Clinical Child Psychologist** Child Psychologists provide expertise in the assessment of children's difficulties to inform diagnosis and work individually with children with a broad range of therapeutic approaches.

➢ **Speech and Language Therapist**: Speech Therapists assess children's speech, language and communication. They provide therapy both individually and in groups. Speech Therapists can facilitate generalisation of skills through indirect therapy with parents and schools.

➢ **Social Worker**: Social Workers work with children and their families in a variety of therapeutic contexts. They also form a valuable link with community care for children who require the input of social services.

➢ **Children's Psychiatric Nurse**: Psychiatric nurses provide a range of services on the team working closely with both children and families. Nursing staff frequently play a role in medication clinics and liaison with school and other agencies.

➢ **Occupational Therapist**: Occupational Therapists assess children's sensory profile and fine and gross motor skills. They also provide therapeutic input to promote motor skill development as indicated.

➢ Other therapists include: family therapists, child psychotherapists and art therapists.

Not all teams have a full complement of staff, but most will include a Child Psychiatrist and Psychiatric Nurse.

What types of therapies may be offered?

Art Therapy: uses the medium of art to explore inner conflicts and to help bring understanding and relief from these difficulties.

Behavioural Therapy: is aimed at changing a child's maladaptive behaviour by rewarding appropriate behaviour.

Cognitive Behavioural Therapy: aims to help young people increase their understanding of how their feelings are linked to thinking patterns and behaviour. Unhelpful patterns of thinking and behaving are targeted which in turn has a positive impact on feelings, behaviour and thinking.

Family Therapy: treats more than one family member in the same session, seeking to explore familial interactions and patterns that may be contributing to the difficulties with which the child presents.

Occupational Therapy: involves the assessment and treatment of motor, sensory and coordination difficulties.

Parenting Training: helps a parent to institute behavioural programmes to change target behaviours. It also focuses on promoting a positive relationship between parent and child.

Play Therapy: uses play with the therapist as a means to exploring the child's difficulties and bringing about their resolution.

Psychodynamic Psychotherapy: seeks to explore unconscious inner conflicts as a means to understand and remediate the child's current difficulties.

Speech and Language Therapy: assesses and treats speech disorders and communication problems.

Supportive Therapy: focuses on the management and resolution of the child's current difficulties focusing on utilizing the child's strengths and available supports.

Resources

Useful Websites

Friends for Life, Booklet. 2007 Barrett & May, www.friendsinfo.net

www.curriculum.edu.au/mindmatters. Curriculum Corporation is a partnership of all Australian Education Ministries. It undertakes activities that are in the national interest and that support and augment the work of the States and Territories in providing educational experiences for all students.

www.aboutourkids.com is the site of The New York Child Study Center.

Bernard, B. 1995. *Fostering Resilience in Children* , California: WestEd. Available online at www.wested.ord/cs/we/view/rs/93

Chapter 1 Introduction

www.rcpsych.ac.uk is the official site of the Royal College of Psychiatrists. It
  contains reading lists for children and teenagers with particular mental health
  difficulties.

www.resilienceproject.org is the official of the International Resilience Research
  Centre

The *Mental Health and Growing Up* series contains 36 factsheets on a range of
  common mental health problems. To order the pack, contact Book Sales at the
  Royal College of Psychiatrists, 17 Belgrave Square, London SW1X 8PG; tel. 020
  7235 2351, ext. 146; fax 020 7245 1231; e-mail booksales@rcpsych.ac.uk or
  you can download them from the above website.

Circulars and Pamphlets

Special Education Circular, SPED 02/05, Special Education Section, Department of
  Education and Science, Cornamaddy, Athlone, Co. Westmeath. August 2005.

Special Education Needs, A Continuum of Support. Resource Pack for Teachers,
  September 2007. Department of Education and Science, Marlborough St.,
  Dublin 1.

Special Education Support Service
Cork Education Support Centre
The Rectory
Western Road
Cork
Tel: 1850 200 0884
Fax: 021 425 5647
Email: info@sess.ie
Website: www.sess.ie

National Educational Psychological Service
24-27 North Frederick Street
Dublin 1
Tel: 01-889 2700
Email: neps@neps.gov.ie

Working Together to make a Difference to Children, National Educational Psychological
  Service. The NEPS model of service available on the Department of Education
  and Science website.

Guidelines Towards a Positive Policy for School Behaviour and Discipline. Circular 20/90, Special Education Section, Department of Education and Science.

Special Educational Needs - A continuum of support, Guidelines for Teachers. National Educational Psychological Service. Department of Education and Science, September 2007

Special Educational Needs - A Continuum of Support, Resource Pack for Teachers, National Educational Psychological Service, Department of Education and Science. September 2007

Books and articles

Stewart, D., Sun, J., Patterson, C., Lemerle, K. & Hardie, M. *Promoting and Building Resilience in Primary School Communities: Evidence form a Comprehensive 'Health Promoting School ' Approach, , The International Journal of Mental health promotion*, vol 6, no.3, August 2004, pp.26-33, The Clifford Beers Foundation.

Benard, B. (1997) *Turning it around for all Youth: From risk to resilience.* New York: Educational resources Information centre (ERIC) Clearinghouse.

Creative Relaxation in Group Work, Tubbs, I.
The Mad, Glad, Sad Game.

McGuire PD. The specialist youth Mental Health model: strengthening the weakest link in the public health system. *Medical Journal of Australia 2007;* 187 (7 suppl): s53-56

Weissberg, RP, Caplan MZ, Sivo,PJ: 'A new conceptual framework for establishing school-based social competence promotion programs', In Bond, L.A and Compas, B.E. (Eds) *Primary prevention and promotion in schools.* Newbury Park, CA: Sage, 1989.

WHO, *Life Skills Education in Schools* (WHO, Division of Mental Health, Geneva) MNH/PSF/93.7, 1993.

Young, I. Williams, T: *The Healthy School.* Scottish Health Education Group, ISBN 0-906323-68-1, Edinburgh, June 1992. Promoting Positive Mental Health.

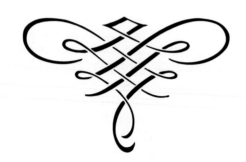

2 Attention Deficit Hyperactivity Disorder (ADHD)

Mark's story

Mark is 9 years old and is constantly in trouble in school. He finds it difficult to sit still in his chair in school and regularly gets up to look out the window. He is easily distracted when taking down his homework from the blackboard and often brings home the wrong books. He has a very short concentration span and this is evident when he is doing his homework or when he is playing games at home. He has difficulty waiting his turn and constantly interrupts when others are talking. He can hardly sit down at mealtimes to eat his meals as he is so energetic and he finds it hard to sit still...

DSM-IV criteria for ADHD

A. Either (1) or (2)

(1) six (or more) of the following symptoms of inattention have persisted for at least six months to a degree that is maladaptive and inconsistent with developmental level:

Inattention

often fails to give close attention to details or makes careless mistakes in school work or other activities

often has difficulty in sustaining attention in tasks or play activities

often does not seem to listen when spoken to directly

often does not follow through on instructions

often has difficulty organising tasks and activities

often avoids, dislikes, or is reluctant to engage in tasks that require sustained mental effort (such as school work or homework)

often loses things necessary for tasks or activities (e.g. toys, school assignments, pencils, books, or tools)

is often easily distracted by extraneous stimuli

is often forgetful in daily activities

(2) six (or more) of the following symptoms of hyperactivity-impulsivity have persisted for at least 6 months to a degree that is maladaptive and inconsistent with developmental level:

Hyperactivity

often fidgets with hands or feet or squirms in seat

often leaves seat in classroom or in other situations in which remaining seated is expected

often runs about or climbs excessively in situations in which it is inappropriate (in adolescents or adults, may be limited to subjective feelings of restlessness)

often has difficulty playing or engaging in leisure activities quietly

is often "on the go" or acts as if "driven by a motor"

often talks excessively

Impulsivity

often blurts out answers before questions have been completed

often has difficulty awaiting turn

often interrupts or intrudes on others (e.g., butts into conversations or games)

B. Some hyperactive-impulsive or inattentive symptoms that cause impairment were present before age of 7 years

C. Some impairment from the symptoms is present in at least two or more settings (e.g., at school [or at work] and at home).

D. There must be clear evidence of clinically significant impairment in social, academic, or occupational functioning.

The symptoms do not occur exclusively during the course of a pervasive developmental disorder and are not better accounted for by another mental disorder (e.g., Mood Disorder, Anxiety Disorder, or a Personality Disorder).

How is the diagnosis of ADHD made?

There are three cardinal symptoms: hyperactivity, impulsivity and attention problems. The symptoms need to be present before the age of 7 years of age, persist for more than 6 months, and be pervasive over time. These symptoms must cause impairment in two or more settings including social situations, school or family and are not due to any other disorder. The core inattention, hyperactivity and impulsive symptoms of the disorder can cause significant impairment in the academic performance and social development of the child and adversely affect functioning within the family.

What are the effects of ADHD?

Children with ADHD may have significant difficulties in the classroom sustaining attention and this may impair their ability to learn.

They often have poor performance and academic failure as a result of uncompleted tasks and not following through instructions.

Many of these children may also have reading difficulties or hand writing difficulties which further compounds their problems.

Children with ADHD may find it difficult to learn social rules easily or to understand social cues. This may have consequences on their capacity to develop friendships which in term impacts negatively on self-esteem and subsequent behaviour.

If children are very impulsive they may find it difficult to take turns while playing games and may interrupt other children while they are talking.

Often children with ADHD find unstructured times such as break time very difficult and they may require assistance during this time.

Is it a serious condition?

If ADHD is untreated there can be very serious consequences in a person's academic, social and family life. School years are particularly difficult for children with ADHD as they have to conform to a style of teaching and educational syllabus which is extremely challenging to children with suboptimal attentional capacity. After finishing school, children have an option to choose study or work in an area where they are more skilled and motivated, hence their existing attention difficulties may not be as impairing or evident.

There is a higher rate of substance misuse and cigarette smoking in teenagers with untreated ADHD. There is also a higher reported incidence of unplanned teenage pregnancies and road traffic accidents in teenagers with untreated ADHD.

How common is ADHD?

ADHD affects 3-5% of school-age children.

There is a 4:1 male to female ratio.

Is ADHD a 'new phenomenon'?

Hippocrates (493 BC) described patients who had "quickened responses to sensory experience, but also less tenaciousness because the soul moves on quickly to the next impression" and attributed this condition to an "overbalance of fire over water". In 1902 the set of symptoms we now recognise as ADHD was called "Morbid Defect of Moral Control" followed by "Encephalitic Behaviour Disorders" in 1922. In 1937 Charles Bradley introduced the use of stimulants to treat hyperactive children. The name "Minimal Brain Disorder" was used in 1960 followed by "Hyperkinetic Reaction" in 1968. In 1980 Dr. Stella Chess described "Hyperactive Child Syndrome" and "Attention Deficit Disorder". In 1987 the disorder was renamed "Attention Deficit Hyperactivity Disorder" by the American Psychiatric Association. It has therefore been around for many decades albeit under many different names.

What causes ADHD?

There is no single cause of ADHD but research has shown that there is a combination of genetic and environmental factors involved. The behavioural and cognitive symptoms of ADHD are thought to be due to an abnormality of dopamine, which is a chemical in the brain. Dopamine is thought to be important in helping us pay attention. When we are concentrating it is released and activates a postsynaptic receptor to create a nerve signal in the brain. This decreases background noise and helps a person to focus. It is thought that children with ADHD are born with a relative deficiency of dopamine. Although dopamine is released it is taken back up too quickly and is not allowed to exert its full effect. As a result there is an increase in background noise and a decrease in focus and attention.

Stimulant medication improves attention by increasing extracellular dopamine in the brain which is believed to increase signal to noise ratio (enhancing task-related neuronal firing) in a part of the brain called the basal ganglia. This is the mechanism for improving attention.

Dopamine also influences motivation and this improves the ability to sustain concentration on tasks by increasing the interest it evokes and thus improving attention and performance.

Genetic Factors

Twin, family and adoption studies have proposed that ADHD can be passed on by genes. In identical twins there is a risk of 80% that they will both develop ADHD. In non-identical twins the rate is approximately 20%. Siblings of children with ADHD have two to three times the risk of having ADHD.

Familial Factors

If the environment at home is disorganised and chaotic this may act as an environmental trigger which, when combined with the child's genetic vulnerability, can exacerbate symptoms of ADHD.

Coexisting Difficulties

Individuals with ADHD often have specific learning disabilities, speech and language disorder, conduct disorder, depression or anxiety symptoms. If a child is struggling academically, it is useful to get a psychological assessment to identify other learning difficulties. A speech and language and occupational therapy assessment may also be required.

What can the teacher do to help?

Children with ADHD need significant support in the classroom setting. The following are guidelines for helping children manage. It is important to provide reassurance and encouragement and focus on any talent or achievements.

Environment

- ➢ Have a few clear organisational/behavioural rules and display them in the classroom;
- ➢ Place the child in the least distracting location away from the door and windows;
- ➢ When giving instructions provide a clear outline of the lesson or topic (standing near a pupil with ADHD can help the child focus);
- ➢ It can be useful to make regular eye contact with the child with ADHD to help focus;
- ➢ Consider seating distractible pupils next to pupils with good study skills and review the arrangement of the desks;
- ➢ Transition times as well as less structured times such as breaks should be closely monitored as children with ADHD can find it difficult to refocus their attention when switching tasks.

Organisation of Teaching

Where possible:

- ➢ Have a daily classroom schedule and establish routines, which are known, predictable and practised;
- ➢ Try to introduce a variety of different topics throughout the lesson as this will help keep distractible children interested;
- ➢ At the end of each class a short summary of the main learning points, can help the child with ADHD to focus;
- ➢ Alternate between reading, writing, drawing and short discussions
- ➢ Use visual aids;
- ➢ Role playing can help children learn historical facts in a fun way;
- ➢ Encourage students to be involved in the lesson and maybe include them in writing on the board;
- ➢ Write simple clear instructions and underline key points. Give assignments one at a time.

Management of Hyperactive/Impulsive symptoms of ADHD in the classroom

- ➢ A restless child could be assigned a task, for example, to write on the blackboard;
- ➢ Allow frequent breaks;
- ➢ Let the child lead certain tasks;

> ➢ Keep the topics varied and use different models of teaching;
> ➢ Working in a pair with a good student;
> ➢ Teach how to 'stop, think, do'.

Management of Inattentive symptoms of ADHD in the classroom

> ➢ Co-operative learning activities;
> ➢ Assign each child in a group a specific role or piece of information that must be shared in the group;
> ➢ Call child by their name before asking them a question;
> ➢ Underline key points to highlight them;
> ➢ Give a warning at the beginning and the end of the teaching session.

Social Skills

> ➢ Model good social skills;
> ➢ Work with parents on agreeing behaviours which need extra attention;
> ➢ Children with ADHD are at risk of peer isolation so it is important to help them integrate with their peers.

Homework

Depending on the child's age:

> ➢ Help the child organise homework notebook and school bag;
> ➢ Have a variety of rewards;
> ➢ Keep track of what work the child has completed and help the child find a system of organising work;
> ➢ Use plenty of praise for assignments done in school and for homework completed;
> ➢ Divide up long assignments into manageable sections and plan with the child when these are due;
> ➢ Help the child develop checklists to ensure the right books are brought home;
> ➢ Use a kitchen timer to indicate periods of independent intense work. This helps a child build up concentration skills gradually.

When is professional help needed?

If the child's symptoms of inattention or hyperactivity and impulsiveness are impairing the child's social, academic and family functioning, then help is required. The child should be brought to a GP to rule out any medical cause for these symptoms. If necessary, hearing and vision should be checked. The child should then be referred to the local CAMHS for a multidisciplinary team assessment.

Treatment

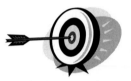 The first stage of treatment is providing education and support, to child and parents, on ADHD and its management. The aim of treatment is to manage the symptoms of ADHD to enable the child to lead a normal life and reach full potential.

Individual

Young people can benefit from extra help in setting up a study timetable. It is also very important that young people are involved in monitoring and making decisions about taking medication.

Family

Parent management training is a fundamental component for all parents. Ruling out ADHD in a parent, helping with home-school liaison and developing consistency at home is part of the process. For families where ADHD has resulted in conflictual relationships developing between children and parents, counselling may be helpful.

Educational

Provide support for any learning difficulties and a structured approach to teaching, as outlined. Teachers can play an important role in helping to monitor the effects of medication and any behaviour strategies that may be useful to help the child.

Medication

> ➤ Medication has been shown to be the most effective intervention for the core symptoms of ADHD;
> ➤ A combined approach of behaviour therapy and medication is the preferred treatment package for children with ADHD and comorbid difficulties;
> ➤ As children develop cognitively they can develop self-monitoring skills to be aware of their difficulties and try to build up their skills to manage their symptoms of ADHD.
> ➤ The medications found effective in ADHD are mostly stimulant medications and their main action is on the Dopamine Pathways in the brain;
> ➤ These medications target symptoms of inattention and hyperactivity/impulsivity. Stimulants should enhance a child's natural abilities, not slow them down or increase hyperactivity;
> ➤ Medication helps focus attention, shut out distraction and allow impulsive children to think before they act;
> ➤ The most common stimulant medication is Methlyphenidate (Ritalin). It works within 20 -30 minutes of being swallowed and lasts for approximately 3 - 4 hours. It is usually prescribed two to three times daily. There are longer acting stimulants Concerta and Ritalin LA which are taken once daily and can last for 8-12 hours. Atomoxetine is also given once a day, lasting 24 hours and is a non-stimulant medication;
> ➤ The common side-effects are reduced appetite and difficulty getting to sleep. Less common side-effects are headaches, tummy pains, tics and irritability. The doctor prescribing medication will give the parents and child information on medication and will monitor it closely. Teachers are a very helpful source in assisting the doctor and family to review the benefits or side-effects of medication.

Essential Fatty acids

Essential fatty acids are found in fish oils. Two important fatty acids are omega 3 and omega 6 fatty acids. Low levels of essential fatty acids are thought to contribute to problems with learning, sleep and temper. Nowadays there are less essential fatty acids in the average diet than previously and many parents like to supplement their children's diet. There are case reports of improvements in some children's attention and concentration when taking supplementary fish oils. A study of young offenders in an institution in Great Britain showed a reduction in violent incidents when a mixture of fish oil, vitamins and minerals was prescribed compared to a group who were given a placebo tablet (a dummy tablet). There is further research required before we can be certain it is useful in children with ADHD, as fish oils can be expensive.

Myths

Children who take Ritalin are more likely to abuse drugs when they are teenagers.
Research has shown that adolescents with untreated ADHD are more likely to abuse illicit drugs.

ADHD only affects behaviour at school.
ADHD affects behaviour in various settings throughout the day, such as at home, at the playground, and during after-school activities. At school, children are most cognitively challenged so it is understandable that their symptoms are most pronounced there. To have a diagnosis of ADHD, a child will also experience some symptoms at home or in other settings.

All children grow out of ADHD
About one third of children's symptoms improve once they reach their teenage years.

Resources

INCADDS is the Irish National Council of ADHD/HKD Support Groups
INCADDDS Member Support Groups Countrywide
HADD Dublin - Carmichael Centre for voluntary groups, Brunswick Street, Dublin 7 Tel: 01-8748349
Clonmel ADHD - 68 Griffith Avenue, Clonmel, Co. Tipperary, Tel: 052-27057
Cork HADD, Kildarra, Bandon, Co. Cork, Tel: 021-4775488
Galway ADHD, Cloon, Claregalway, Co. Galway, Tel: 091-98266
Kilkenny ADHD, Jerpoint Abbey, Thomastown, Co. Kilkenny, Tel: 056-54954
    www.nimh.nih.gov/health/topics/attention-deficit-hyperactivity-disorder-adhd

Chapter 2

Reading Resources

Attention/Deficit Hyperactivity Disorder - A Practical Guide for Teachers. Cooper, S and Ideus, C, .

A Parent's Guide to Attention Deficit Disorders. New York: Dell Publishing, 1991.

Attention Deficit Hyperactivity Disorder: A multidisciplinary approach. Henry K. Holowenko, Jessica Kingsley, London

ADD: Practical activities in school. Tony Attwood.

Attention, Please!: A comprehensive Guide for Successfully Parenting Children with Attention Disorders and Hyperactivity. Atlanta, GA:SPI: Press, 1991.

Maybe you know my kid: A Parent's Guide to Identifying, Understanding, and Helping your Child with ADHD. New York: Birch Lane Press ,1990

Taking Charge of ADHD, Russell Barkley. Guildford Press, 1995.

Understanding ADHD by Christopher Green, Vermilion, 1994.

The Hyperactive Child, a Parent's Guide by Professor Eric Taylor (Vermilion 1994).

The ADHD Handbook - For Parents and Professionals by Dr. Alison Munden and Dr. Jon Arcleus.

Hyperactivity Why Won't My Child Pay Attention? Complete Guide to ADD for parents, teachers and health care professionals by Dr's Sam and Michael Goldstein.

For Children Eagle Eyes: A Child's View of Attention Deficit Disorder, by Jeanne Gehret, M.A. For ages 5+.

Learning to Slow down and Pay Attention - A book for kids about ADD. By Kathleen G. Nadeau, Ph.D and Ellen B. Dixon, Ph.D.

Putting on the Brakes by Patricia Quinn M.D. & Judith Stern M.A. for ages 8-12.

Shelley The Hyperactive Turtle by Deborah Moss for ages 3-7

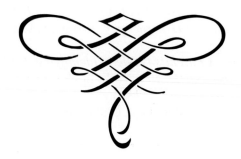

3 Anxiety Disorders

Jake's story

Jake is a fifteen-year-old boy and is an only child. He has always been shy but previously had enjoyed the company of a small group of friends. Recently, Jake has become increasingly conscious of blushing in public. He feels that all his peers have noticed this. He is missing an increasing number of days from school. He tells his mother that he doesn't want to read in front of the class or have lunch with classmates believing he will 'make a fool' of himself. Jake is becoming increasingly limited in the activities he is willing to engage in. Consequently, he is becoming socially isolated leading to numerous rows with his father who feels he should 'just get on with it'…

Introduction

Anxiety is an unpleasant but normal emotion, which is a universal experience. Anxiety has a number of components including the emotion itself, physiological aspects (such as butterflies in the stomach, palpitations, shaking hands) and cognitive aspects that include the thoughts evoked by the anticipation of the undesirable experience.

Anxiety disorders represent an extreme manifestation of normal anxiety and occur when the anxiety system becomes dysregulated. Consequently, children with anxiety disorders experience anxiety as an overwhelming emotion, which has a significant impact on their day-to-day lives. It can limit a child's life in any or all spheres including home-life, school, interactions with peers and social activities.

The Development of Fears

Stranger Anxiety is typically the first fear that an infant displays and is developmentally normal between the ages of about seven to eighteen months. Infants shows signs of fear or distress in the presence of an unknown person especially if they are not in close proximity to a familiar care-giver. This fear usually decreases at approximately two years of age. Fears follow a typical developmental pathway as outlined below:

Table 3.1   Development of Fears

7-18 months	Stranger Anxiety
7-18 months:	Separation Anxiety
Infants:	Heights, loud noises, loss of physical support
1-3 years:	Strangers & loud noises
5-7 years:	Animals, darkness, monsters
Adolescence	Exams, health, abilities, sexual matters, personal performance

Separation Anxiety is also very common in infants and develops at a similar age to stranger anxiety, peaking at about fifteen to eighteen months. If the child is securely attached, this fear decreases after the age of two or three as the child is able to predict the return of their primary care-giver. Separation

Anxiety only becomes a disorder if it persists after three years of age and is accompanied by persistent and pervasive fears.

How are Anxiety Disorders diagnosed?

There are a number of specific anxiety disorders including:
- ➢ Specific phobias;
- ➢ Selective Mutism;
- ➢ Separation Anxiety Disorder;
- ➢ Generalised Anxiety Disorder;
- ➢ Social Phobia;
- ➢ Panic Disorder with or without agoraphobia;
- ➢ Obsessive Compulsive Disorder is classified as an anxiety disorder but is covered in a separate chapter.

Note: School refusal is not a specific anxiety disorder diagnosis. In fact, a child may refuse to attend school as a result of the above disorders and indeed many other reasons that have nothing to do with anxiety.

Specific Phobias

DSM-IV Criteria for Specific Phobias

- Marked and persistent fear that is excessive or unreasonable, cued by the presence or anticipation of a specific object or situation (e.g., flying, heights, animals, receiving an injection, seeing blood).
- Exposure to the phobic stimulus almost invariably provokes an immediate anxiety response, which may take the form of a situationally bound or situationally predisposed Panic Attack (see definition section 5). Note: In children, the anxiety may be expressed by crying, tantrums, freezing, or clinging.
- The person recognizes that the fear is excessive or unreasonable. Note: In children, this feature may be absent.
- The phobic situation(s) is (are) avoided or else is endured with intense anxiety or distress.
- The avoidance, anxious anticipation, or distress in the feared situation(s) interferes significantly with the person's normal routine, occupational (or academic) functioning, or social activities or relationships, or there is marked distress about having the phobia.
- In individuals under age 18 years, the duration is at least 6 months.

Almost 10% of children have specific phobias. Common childhood fears include fear of certain animals, insects, the dark, thunder, blood and injections. If the fear is persistent, intense and disabling, then the fear has reached phobic proportions. Children with specific phobias may not recognise that their fears are excessive or unrealistic.

The specific type of phobia can be specified as follows:

Animal Type;

Natural Environment Type (e.g., heights, storms, water);

Blood-Injection-Injury Type;

Situational Type (e.g., aeroplanes, lifts, enclosed places);

Other Type (e.g., phobic avoidance of situations that may lead to choking, vomiting, or contracting an illness; in children, avoidance of loud sounds or costumed characters).

Selective Mutism

Selective Mutism is conceptualised as a subtype of social phobia which occurs in children. The disorder is characterised by a failure to speak in certain situations such as the classroom while speaking freely with close friends and family members in the home environment. There may also be other anxiety symptoms present which require treatment.

DSM-IV Criteria for Selective Mutism

- Consistent failure to speak in specific social situations (in which there is an expectation for speaking, e.g., at school) despite speaking in other situations.
- The disturbance interferes with educational or occupational achievement or with social communication.
- The duration of the disturbance is at least 1 month (not limited to the first month of school).
- The failure to speak is not due to a lack of knowledge of, or comfort with, the spoken language required in the social situation.
- The disturbance is not better accounted for by a Communication Disorder (e.g., Stuttering) and does not occur exclusively during the course of a Pervasive Development Disorder, Schizophrenia, or other Psychotic Disorder.

Selective Mutism is more common than previously thought. One Irish study suggested a prevalence rate of 700/100,000 (ref. at end of chapter). It is more common in immigrant children where English is not their first language, in twins, in socially isolated families, or in families who have other anxiety disorders.

Separation Anxiety Disorder

Approximately 4% of children meet diagnostic criteria for separation anxiety disorder. This is characterised by developmentally inappropriate and excessive fear following the actual or potential separation from the child's attachment figure (usually the mother). Typically it manifests itself as anxious avoidance of school or other situations where the child may be separated from the primary caregiver. The child displays distress with separation and typically harbours fears as to the safety of parents in their absence. The child may describe fears that parents will be kidnapped, involved in a car crash or become severely ill.

DSM IV Criteria for Separation Anxiety Disorder

1) Developmentally inappropriate and excessive anxiety concerning separation from home or from those to whom the individual is attached, as evidenced by three (or more) of the following:
   - recurrent excessive distress when separation from home or major attachment figures occurs or is anticipated
   - persistent and excessive worry about losing, or about possible harm befalling, major attachment figures
   - persistent and excessive worry that an untoward event will lead to separation from a major attachment figure (e.g., getting lost or being kidnapped)
   - persistent reluctance or refusal to go to school or elsewhere because of fear of separation
   - persistently and excessively fearful or reluctant to be alone or without major attachment figures at home or without significant adults in other settings
   - persistent reluctance or refusal to go to sleep without being near a major attachment figure or to sleep away from home
   - repeated nightmares involving the theme of separation
   - repeated complaints of physical symptoms (such as headaches, stomachaches, nausea, or vomiting) when separation from major attachment figures occurs or is anticipated

2) The duration of the disturbance is at least 4 weeks.
3) The onset is before age 18 years

Generalised Anxiety Disorder

The prevalence of generalised anxiety in children is approximately 4.5%. For children with generalised anxiety, the disorder is characterised by almost daily worry about numerous things such as schoolwork, how they are perceived by friends and the well-being of family members. In order to be diagnosed with this condition, the child's worry must be excessive, longer than six months in duration and cause distress or impairment in functioning in school or at home.

DSM-IV Criteria for Generalised Anxiety Disorder

- Excessive anxiety and worry (apprehensive expectation), occurring more days than not for at least 6 months, about a number of events or activities (such as work or school performance).
- The person finds it difficult to control the worry.
- The anxiety and worry are associated with three (or more) of the following six symptoms (with at least some symptoms present for more days than not for the past 6 months). Note: Only one item is required in children.
- restlessness or feeling keyed up or on edge
- being easily fatigued
- difficulty concentrating or mind going blank
- irritability
- muscle tension
- sleep disturbance (difficulty falling or staying asleep, or restless unsatisfying sleep)

The anxiety, worry, or physical symptoms cause clinically significant distress or impairment in social, occupational, or other important areas of functioning.

Reprinted with permission from The Diagnostic and Statistical Manual of Mental Disorders, Text Revision, Fourth Edition, (Copyright 2000). American Psychiatric Association.

Social Phobia

Social Phobia is rare before puberty and about 1% of children may have disabling symptoms. The disorder is characterised by an intense fear of situations where the child perceives he will be scrutinised by others. These situations may include eating in the canteen, parties and group activities. Ultimately, these situations are avoided and the young person may become increasingly isolated.

DSM-IV Criteria for Social Phobia

- A marked and persistent fear of one or more social or performance situations in which the person is exposed to unfamiliar people or to possible scrutiny by others. The individual fears that he or she will act in a way (or show anxiety symptoms) that will be humiliating or embarrassing.
  Note: In children, there must be evidence of the capacity for age–appropriate social relationships with familiar people and the anxiety must occur in peer settings, not just in interactions with adults.
- Exposure to the feared social situation almost invariably provokes anxiety, which may take the form of a situationally bound or situationally predisposed Panic Attack.
  Note: In children, the anxiety may be expressed by crying, tantrums, freezing, or shrinking from social situations with unfamiliar people.
- The person recognizes that the fear is excessive or unreasonable. Note: In children, this feature may be absent.
- The feared social or performance situations are avoided or else are endured with intense anxiety or distress.
- The avoidance, anxious anticipation, or distress in the feared social or performance situation(s) interferes significantly with the person's normal routine, occupational (academic) functioning, or social activities or relationships, or there is marked distress about having the phobia.
- In individuals under age 18 years, the duration is at least 6 months.

Panic Disorder with or without Agoraphobia

Panic disorder is rare prior to puberty but can occur. The onset of panic disorder does not reach its peak incidence until adulthood. It is characterised by a series of panic attacks i.e. sudden onset of anxiety associated with physical symptoms such as difficulty breathing or palpitations. The attack is frequently associated with a belief that the young person is about to die. The individual becomes increasingly anxious about the possibility of further unprovoked attacks and may be in a constant state of heightened anxiety in between panic attacks.

DSM-IV Criteria for Panic Disorder with or without Agoraphobia

A)   Recurrent unexpected Panic Attacks and at least one of the attacks has been followed by one month (or more) of one (or more) of the following:

- (1) persistent concern about having additional attacks
- (2) worry about the implications of the attack or its consequences (e.g., losing control, having a heart attack, "going crazy")
- (3) a significant change in behaviour related to the attacks

B.   The presence of Agoraphobia
Definition: A Panic Attack is defined as: A discrete period of intense fear or discomfort, in which four (or more) of the following symptoms developed abruptly and reached a peak within 10 minutes:

- (1) palpitations, pounding heart, or accelerated heart rate
- (2) sweating
- (3) trembling or shaking
- (4) sensations of shortness of breath or smothering
- (5) feeling of choking
- (6) chest pain or discomfort
- (7) nausea or abdominal distress
- (8) feeling dizzy, unsteady, lightheaded, or faint
- (9) derealization (feelings of unreality) or depersonalization (being detached from oneself)
- (10) fear of losing control or going crazy
- (11) fear of dying
- (12) paresthesias (numbness or tingling sensations)
- (13) chills or hot flushes

Agoraphobia

Agoraphobia is defined as anxiety about being in places or situations from which escape might be difficult (or embarrassing) or in which help may not be available in the event of having a Panic Attack. Agoraphobic fears typically involve characteristic clusters of situations that include being outside the home alone; being in a crowd or standing in a queue; being on a bridge; and travelling in a bus, train, or car.

The situations are avoided (e.g., travel is restricted) or else are endured with marked distress or anxiety about having a Panic Attack, or require the presence of a companion.

What are the signs of Anxiety Disorders?

The experience of anxiety is very subjective. Therefore, the objective reports of teachers are very important in assessing the overall impact and severity of the disorder.

Signs may include:

➢ Excessive worrying;
➢ Fear of being separated from parents;
➢ Difficulty going in or staying in school;
➢ Avoiding specific places or situations;
➢ Difficulty with reading aloud in class, performing in sports, public speaking;
➢ Extreme shyness or self-consciousness;
➢ May appear very tired due to difficulty sleeping;
➢ Poor concentration;
➢ Crying easily;
➢ Repeated physical complaints such as headaches and stomach-aches;
➢ Breathlessness;
➢ Appearing tense, fidgety, using the toilet often;
➢ Lack of interest in peer activities;
➢ Dread of unstructured time with peers;
➢ Dread of social or performance situations;
➢ Panic attacks;
➢ Appearing isolated and not part of peer group;
➢ Often alone during break time or other unstructured sessions.

Can anyone develop an Anxiety Disorder?

As a group, Anxiety Disorders are one of the commonest psychological difficulties experienced by young people and can potentially develop in any child or young person. The prevalence rate is between five and twenty per cent.

Table 3.2   Prevalence of Anxiety Disorders

Specific Phobias:	9.2%
Separation Anxiety Disorder:	4.1%
Generalised Anxiety Disorder:	4.6%
Social Phobias:	1%

What are the effects of Anxiety Disorders?

Anxiety can be very distressing. In order to minimise distress, children may increasingly try to avoid situations which they find difficult such as school or other social interaction. Consequently, the child may become increasingly isolated and withdrawn from age-appropriate activities. The child may also become increasingly irritable and, in some cases, depressed.

Are Anxiety Disorders serious conditions?

Anxiety Disorders can have long-term consequences for children and teenagers, particularly if they do not receive treatment. A child may live a very restricted lifestyle due to anxiety symptoms. The child's inability to tolerate anxiety can have a negative impact in adult life in terms of the person's ability to cope with the challenges of new situations and social demands. These disorders may occur again in adulthood in a similar way or the person may develop a different range of symptoms. For example, the child who is selectively mute may go on to develop social phobia in adulthood.

What causes Anxiety Disorders?

As with almost all mental health difficulties, the causes are multiple and these risk factors interact in a complex way. Anxiety Disorders are thought to arise from the interplay between psychological, biological and social factors.

Biological

Some research has suggested that chemicals in the brain such as serotonin and noradrenaline have an important role in the development of anxiety disorders. Some children may be born with relative deficiencies of some chemicals leading to increased vulnerability to experiencing anxiety. However, the way in which these chemicals interact with other risk factors has yet to be established.

Studies of families and identical twins (who share the same genetic make-up) suggest that there is a genetic component to these disorders.

Temperament

Temperamental factors (inborn personality traits) have also been linked to the development of anxiety disorders in children. For example, 50% of children who display the trait of Behavioural Inhibition will go on to develop some sort of anxiety disorder. Behavioural Inhibition refers to a characteristic cluster of behaviours, which are displayed when the child is faced with an unfamiliar situation or person. Behavioural Inhibition is an early temperamental trait that can be seen in toddlers. The toddler who displays Behavioural Inhibition stops what they are doing when they notice an unfamiliar person or situation and typically becomes disconcerted moving around, crying and becoming irritable. Longitudinal studies (which follow children over prolonged periods) have established that Behavioural Inhibition is an enduring character trait. Children of parents with anxiety or depression are more likely to display Behavioural Inhibition.

Research also suggests that children who are innately shy are more at risk of developing anxiety disorders. Other personality types that have been linked with the development of Anxiety Disorders include those displaying perfectionistic and avoidant traits.

Family Factors

Children who have a less secure attachment with their mothers or primary caregiver are at increased risk of developing anxiety disorders. It has also been shown that anxiety and phobic disorders can be learned through direct observation of other people such as parents (parental modelling). It may seem unsurprising therefore that anxiety disorders often run in families. However, the complex interplay between genes, brain chemicals, innate temperament and learned behaviours is not well understood.

What can the teacher do to help?

Help!

Building up the child's confidence and self-esteem is key. Selectively attend to tasks that are accomplished by the child no matter how small. Use liberal praise for anything the child manages or is good at.

Model how to behave in anxiety-provoking situations by giving explicit instructions. For example, telling the child "when you do not know the answer move on to the next question".

Try to decrease the stress associated with school situations. For example, if distressed by reading to the whole class, allow the student to read to small groups or individually or if practicable into a tape-recorder. Give such students adequate notice of a change in routine and give them an alternative focus when an anxiety-provoking situation is imminent. For example, ask the child to collect the copy books.

Discuss any issues around the child's response to stress in private. Try to facilitate discussions with the student which emphasise the child's progress. For example, highlight specific situations that the child is now able to handle. Similarly, try to pinpoint with the child any specific obstacles that are preventing progress. Help to gently challenge the student's assumptions. For example, if the child describes being worried about not being accepted or included by peers, ask the child who is happy to see them in the morning.

Help the child to challenge his own anxiety-provoking thoughts with more constructive alternatives. For example, if the child fears crying when entering the school yard ask what could be done before the crying starts - 'can you read something that makes you laugh, play a game of chase etc.'Or ask:

'...did you ever come into school and not cry, what did you do that day...'

If you become concerned about a child in your class, discuss this with parents so that they too can begin to help to develop the child's self-confidence and challenge fears.

When is professional help required?

For some children, parental and teacher support will be insufficient to allow them overcome their anxiety. If a student's anxiety symptoms are causing distress or are having a significant negative impact on his or her day-to-day functioning, parents should be advised to have their child assessed by their GP. The GP will then decide if referral to the CAMHs is required.

Treatment

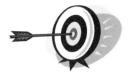

If a child has severe symptoms of anxiety, referral to CAMHS is required. Firstly, the child will have a thorough assessment to detail the nature of the fears and worries and to establish whether these fears are developmentally appropriate. The evaluation will explore how long the child has been having these difficulties and the steps that have been taken to alleviate them. The assessment will also highlight the impact the anxiety is having on the child's ability to function in different situations. Consideration will also be given to any situations or people in the child's life who are unconsciously maintaining the anxiety. For example, a mother who is becoming highly anxious when separating from her child at the school gates may inadvertently increase her child's anxiety. She may then be very quick to let her child stay at home from school reinforcing the child's self-perception of inability to cope with stress. This in turn confirms to the child that avoidance is the best way to cope with anxiety provoking situations.

Different therapeutic approaches will be necessary depending on the specific Anxiety Disorder with which the child presents and any associated problems. Treatment leads to reduction or resolution of symptoms in up to 70-90% of young people. However, the underlying vulnerability to anxiety frequently remains and may present again in adulthood as different types of anxiety symptoms or disorders.

Some of the most common treatments are:

Cognitive Behavioural Therapy (CBT)
Research has established that CBT is a very effective treatment for Anxiety Disorders. CBT encompasses a number of different approaches to help the child conquer anxiety. The initial steps usually focus on helping the child to understand more about the nature of anxiety and to understand that anxiety itself is a normal and common feeling. It is very important for the child to understand that there is a physiological basis to anxiety and that simple relaxation exercises (such as deep breaths) can decrease anxious feelings. It is essential that parents too are helped to develop this awareness.

Another core component of the treatment is helping the child to develop more realistic cognitions about anxiety provoking situations. Finally behavioural 'experiments' are designed with the child in a step-wise format. This allows the child to break down feared situations into a number of smaller more manageable steps. This graded approach allows the child to face fears in a structured and supported way.

Medication

Medication may be required depending on the nature and severity of the symptoms. Medication may also be required for children whose symptoms do not improve with CBT. The medications most commonly used are Selective Serotonin Reuptake Inhibitors (SSRIs). The most frequently used SSRI is Fluoxetine (Prozac). If medication is used parents will be given information on side effects and the medication will be carefully monitored. The teacher may be asked to give feedback on effectiveness of the medication and on any side-effects.

Combination Treatments

Combination treatments involve both medication and therapy. This can be a very effective treatment approach when the child is severely distressed or not responding as desired to one or other approach independently.

Myths

This is just a phase

Everyone goes through times in their life when they have more worries than at other stages. However, anxiety disorders are qualitatively different to these 'phases'. When a child has an anxiety disorder, worries are overwhelming to the child and significantly limit the child's capacity to be involved in routine daily activities.

Avoiding anxiety provoking situations is helpful

Allowing the child to avoid situations which are anxiety provoking only serves to maintain the problem. This confirms the child's self perception of being unable to cope and feeds into a sense of helplessness. It is better to allow the child to experience the feared situations with support and master how to overcome the fear.

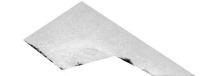

Chapter 3 Anxiety Disorders

To resolve anxiety symptoms it is essential to know how and why they started

For the majority of children, it is much more helpful to start with the 'here and now', helping the child to understand that anxiety is normal and supporting them to allow them to experience anxiety provoking situations. Searching for a cause to a particular anxiety often does not yield any results.

Anxiety Disorders are part of a child's personality and can not be changed

Anxiety Disorders occur when normal anxiety becomes dysregulated. Anxiety Disorders respond very well to treatments including Cognitive Behavioural Therapy, medication or a combination of both.

Resources

Anxiety Disorders in Children and Adolescents. J. S. March Guilford 1995

Elective Mutism Manual: a guide for parents, teachers, clinicians and the child. Louise Sharkey, Fiona McNicholas and Maire Begley. (Available free while in stock from the Lucena Foundation, 59 Orwell Road, Rathgar, Dublin 6. €5 for postage)

Worried No More: Help and Hope for Anxious Children. Aureen Pinto Wagner, Ph.D. Lighthouse Press, Inc. 2002

Helping Your Anxious child: A Step-by-Step Guide for Parents. Ronald Rapee, Ph.D., Susan H. Spence, Ph.D., Vanessa Cobham, Ph.D. and Ann Wignall New Harbinger Publications, Inc. 2000

Keys to Parenting Your Anxious Child. Katharine Manassis M.D. Barron's Educational Series, Inc. 1996

Clinical Handbook of Anxiety Disorders in Children and Adolescents. A. Eisen et al (Eds.) Jason Aronson 1995

Monsters Under the Bed and Other Childhood Fears: Helping Your Child Overcome Anxieties, Fears, and Phobias. S.W. Garber, M.D. Garber, & R.F. Spitzman Villard Books 1993

r Children:

Into the Great Forest: A Story for Children Away from Parents for the First Time, I.W. Marcus & P. Marcus.Magination Press 1992

Night Light: A Story for Children Afraid of the Dark. J. Dutro. Magination Press 1991

Anxiety Disorders

Anxiety Disorders Association of America. www.adaa.org
Mental Health Association of New York city. Helping Children Handle Disaster-Related Anxiety. www.mhaofnyc.org/

National Institute of Mental Health. www.nimh.nih.gov/healthinformation/anxietymenu.cfm

Temple University Child & Adolescent Anxiety Disorders Clinic. www.childanxiety.org

Irish Prevalence Study. Selective Mutism Manual - available upon request to Lucena Clinic, Rathgar, Dublin.

4 Autistic Spectrum Disorders

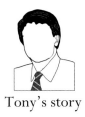

Tony's story

Tony is a 10 year old boy who has a fascination with trains. As a toddler he loved 'Thomas the Tank Engine' and talked about him all the time. Now he collects miniature trains and train timetables. He watched all the DVDs with stories about trains that he could and he learned all the words off verbatim. When anyone calls to the house he talks to them at length about trains. He seems to find it hard to make friends as he always wants to play games his way and finds it difficult to take turns. He often feels that the other children are teasing him and misinterprets comments that they make to him. When his teacher asks him questions in class he often gives the completely wrong answer and frequently offers interesting but nonessential information on trains to her. Despite being Irish he speaks with an American accent in a very precise way and does not seem to understand jokes that other people make...

What is Autism and Asperger's Syndrome?

Autism is a pervasive developmental disorder characterised by difficulties in communication, difficulties in the development of reciprocal social relationships and restricted, stereotyped interests. These developmental abnormalities must have been present in the first three years of life for the diagnosis to be made. It was first described by Leo Kanner in 1943 as: "Abnormal development of social reciprocity, abnormal development of language, especially as it is used for communicating with other persons, and desire for sameness, as seen in repetitive rituals or intense circumscribed interests." Autism is a life-long disorder and although appropriate intervention can improve the outcome, some of the basic deficits persist. Autistic Spectrum Disorders (ASDs) are described across many ethnic groups and different cultures.

Autism is now seen as a disorder of the developing brain, mainly genetic in origin and part of a wider spectrum of disorders. The Autistic Spectrum ranges from children who meet criteria for Autism and have no language to children with normal development of structural language but who have difficulties with social communication and rigid, stereotyped interests (Asperger's Syndrome).

Asperger's Syndrome was first described by Hans Asperger in 1944 when he coined the term "Autistic psychopathy". This is now known as Asperger's Syndrome. Children with Asperger's Syndrome often have normal intelligence and language development but make inappropriate social approaches. They often have good grammar and vocabulary, but can only talk about a narrow range of special interests. They often show resistance to change and abnormalities of motor coordination. Those with Asperger's Syndrome have a better outcome in later life, achieving greater levels of independence and social functioning. The child's overall prognosis is determined by language ability, cognitive level, overall level of behavioural disturbance and adaptive functioning. Children with Asperger's Syndrome often have significant deficits in social skills but can be very successful academically. About 50% of children with Autism acquire speech but if there is no speech by the age of 5 it is unlikely to develop. Ten per cent of adults with Autism work and live independently. A poor prognosis is associated with lack of language development and an IQ of less than 60.

Impairments in Children with ASD

Children with ASD have difficulty in 3 main areas: social interaction, communication and a narrow range of repetitive activities and behaviour. Impairment in social interaction is evident through a lack of joint attention (such as when a parent unsuccessfully attempts to draw the child's attention to something) and deficits in meaningful eye contact. Children with ASD may seem to ignore other people's feelings or may appear insensitive to other people's needs. Children may find it hard to express their emotions verbally or nonverbally. They often lack the ability to think of other people's point of view and to understand and predict the actions of others. Children with Autism often have difficulty making and keeping friends.

Children with Autism are often preoccupied with preferred interests and may be unaware of social cues in the environment. For example, they will talk in detail about one of their favourite topics, not noticing that the listener is uninterested. Children can also have difficulties with symbolic play (using one object to represent another object).

Impairments in communication include language delay or lack of language, impaired conversational skills, learnt phrases, repetitive or made-up language and lack of pretend play. The semantic and pragmatic use of language is difficult for children with ASD. A child with ASD may have difficulty in establishing a two-way conversation and keeping the conversation going. The child is less likely to start a social conversation unless it is about a favourite interest such as the train timetable. The child's conversation may consist of a monologue rather than a social conversation. There may be abnormalities of pitch and intonation. Socializing with other children may be particularly hard. Adults are more likely than other children to make allowances for the child and can keep conversation going if they detect that the child is struggling. They may misinterpret others, i.e. think that someone is making fun of them. They may be very sensitive to comments made to them. They may interpret requests literally (e.g. "pull up your socks").

Children with ASD prefer routine and can be very resistant to change. This can have a significant impact on the child's family and the child can become extremely distressed if some unexpected change occurs at home or in school. Children with Autism may stick rigidly to a daily timetable and classroom rules. They may need a certain routine and to do things in a particular order to avoid becoming distressed. They may sit in the same seat, travel the same

DSM IV criteria for Autistic Disorder

A.   A total of six or more items from (1), (2), and (3), with at least two from (1), and one each from (2) and (3).

(1) qualitative impairment in social interaction, as manifested by at least two of the following:
- marked impairment in the use of multiple nonverbal behaviours such as eye to eye gaze, facial expression, body postures, and gestures to regulate social interaction.
- failure to develop peer relationships appropriate to developmental level
- a lack of spontaneous seeking to share enjoyment, interest, or achievements with other people (e.g., by a lack of showing, bringing or pointing out objects of interest)
- lack of social or emotional reciprocity

(2) qualitative impairments in communication as manifested by at least one of the following:
- (a) delay in, or total lack of, the development of spoken language (not accompanied by an attempt to compensate through alternative modes of communication such as gesture or mime).
- (b) in individuals with adequate speech, marked impairment in the ability to initiate or sustain a conversation with others.
- (c) stereotyped and repetitive use of language or idiosyncratic language
- (d) lack of varied, spontaneous make believe or social imitative play appropriate to developmental level.

(3) restricted repetitive and stereotyped patterns of behaviour, interests, and activities, as manifested by at least one of the following:
- encompassing preoccupation with one or more stereotyped and restricted patterns of interest that is abnormal either in intensity or focus.
- apparently inflexible adherence to specific, non-functional routines or ritual.
- stereotyped and repetitive motor mannerisms (e.g., hand or finger flapping or twisting, or complex whole body movements).
- persistent preoccupation with parts of objects.

B. Delays or abnormal functioning in at least one of the following areas, with onset prior to age 3 years: (1) social interaction, 2) language as used in social communication, or (3) symbolic or imaginative play.

C. The disturbance is not better accounted for by Rett's Disorder or Childhood Disintegrative Disorder.

route to school and unpack their bag in a particular order. Some children with Autism play with unusual objects or develop an obsessive interest in one particular type of toy (e.g. dinosaurs or robots).

Children with ASD can be very sensitive to their environment. They may become uncomfortable in crowded places and can be sensitive to certain noises and may put their hands over their ears. Sometimes they can appear deaf as they may ignore the human voice or may focus on other noises. Children with ASD may also be sensitive to the sensation of certain materials on their skin and often protest about wearing certain types of clothes.

DSM IV criteria for Asperger's Disorder

A.   Qualitative impairment in social interaction, as manifested by at least two of the following:

- marked impairment in the use of multiple nonverbal behaviours such as eye-to-eye gaze, facial expression, body postures, and gestures to regulate social interaction
- failure to develop peer relationships appropriate to developmental level
- a lack of spontaneous seeking to share enjoyment, interests, or achievements with other people (e.g., by a lack of showing, bringing, or pointing out objects of interest to other people)
- lack of social or emotional reciprocity

B.   Restricted repetitive and stereotyped patterns of behaviour, interests, and activities, as manifested by at least one of the following:

- (1) encompassing preoccupation with one or more stereotyped and restricted patterns of interest that is abnormal either in intensity or focus.
- (2) apparently inflexible adherence to specific, non-functional routines or ritual.
- stereotyped and repetitive motor mannerisms (e.g., hand or finger flapping or twisting, or complex whole body movements).
- persistent preoccupation with parts of objects.

C.   The disturbance causes clinically significant impairment in social, occupational, or other important areas of functioning.

D.   There is no clinically significant general delay in language (e.g., single use words by age 2 years, communicative phrases used by age 3 years.)

Reprinted with permission from The Diagnostic and Statistical Manual of Mental Disorders, Text Revision, Fourth Edition, (Copyright 2000). American Psychiatric Association.

How common is Autistic Spectrum Disorder?

Table 4.1   Prevalence of Autistic Spectrum Disorder

1/1000	in the general population for core Autism
1/250-500	Asperger's Syndrome
3/100	if one person in the family has Autistic Spectrum Disorder
3/10	if a sibling has ASD

Are Autistic Spectrum Disorders a new phenomenon?

There are accounts describing the 'Wild boy of Aveyron' who was a 12 year-old living wild in the woods of south-central France at the end of the 18th century. He was captured and placed under the care of a physician called J.M. Itard. Itard wrote long accounts of the boy's behaviour which are very similar to what we now call Autism.

What causes Autistic Spectrum Disorders?

Research suggests that in many cases ASD is a genetically based brain disorder that develops during the first few weeks of foetal growth and that many different genes are involved.

Genetic Theories

In twin studies with identical twins there is a 91% chance of both having Autism. In non-identical twins there is a 30% chance of both twins having an ASD. This shows that there is a strong genetic component involved but that there are also other factors contributing to inheriting Autism.

Studies that have explored Autism in families have established that frequently a number of members of the same family may show varying levels of autistic traits; for example one child may have classic Autism, the child's father may have undiagnosed Asperger's Syndrome and an uncle may have autistic behaviours which do not reach full diagnostic criteria. If a family has one child with Autism, there is a 3% chance that they could have another child with either Autism or Asperger's Syndrome.

Psychological Theories

Psychological theories suggest that the child with Autism is born with an 'inborn error' in the ability to communicate and relate to others. This suggests that children with Autism are less able to respond to social or emotional information such as tone of voice than to non-social input such as a train whistle.

Theory of Mind

This hypothesis suggests that normally developing children can recognise various facial expressions at around five months and understanding the meaning of such expressions (theory of mind) occurs a few months later. Children begin to apply non-verbal information to guide behaviour once they understand non-verbal expressions. However, children with ASD have difficulties with this and as a result affects their ability both to think of other people's point of view and to understand and predict actions.

Other Theories

There are many other theories postulated that do not have significant scientific basis. One such theory is the 'leaky bowel theory'. This theory suggests that peptides leak across the bowel mucosa and across the blood-brain barrier causing autistic symptoms. Gluten and casein free diet are suggested to reduce autistic symptoms. This has not been proven scientifically and it is very important that children are not undernourished if parents are following a restricted diet plan with their child.

It is also important to note that there are a number of theories about Autism which have no basis in science. One such theory which has been conclusively disproved is that Autism is caused by the Measles, Mumps and Rubella vaccine (MMR). This false conclusion was based on one study in 2001 by Furlano which found measles gene material in bowel biopsies taken from individuals with Autism and Irritable Bowel Disorder. It is clear that when the MMR vaccine was introduced for all children, there was no associated increase in cases of Autism. Also it is worth noting that if children are not vaccinated with the MMR and are exposed to measles or rubella they may end up with Autistic like symptoms as a serious side-effect.

What can the teacher do to help?

Children with Autism do best in a well-structured educational environment with experienced teachers.

A structured regime of behaviour training may improve a child's communication and social skills. It is important that only one behaviour is targeted at a time. The first step is to reduce any specific problems such as aggression or self-injury. As the child is challenged to change behaviour, problems may initially escalate prior to objective improvement. It is essential to persevere if the programme is to be successful. Programmes need to be individualised for each child to respond to particular challenges. Research has concluded that the most successful programmes are those that are planned and agreed between teachers and parents. This ensures that the child receives very consistent messages and that the environment is very responsive to particular needs.

Children with ASD are vulnerable to bullying and teasing in school. It is important that teachers look out for this and intervene straight away if a bullying incident occurs. It is important to utilise the child's special skills or interests to learn and develop self-esteem and encourage all pro-social behaviour. For example, if the child with ASD has a special interest in computers and is allowed to demonstrate this special skill to the class, self-confidence will be increased as will positive feedback and interaction with peers.

The child will also need assistance to understand certain socially complicated situations. It is important to avoid using sarcasm or double meanings or certain proverbs, as the child may struggle to understand them and may take the words literally. If using this type of language, use it as an opportunity to explain the meaning to the child.

When is professional help needed?

If you suspect a child has features of ASD, it is important to discuss this with parents. If the child is struggling socially or academically, consider advising parents of the benefit of referral to a professional for diagnosis. For children with significant language difficulties, an assessment by a speech and language therapist is required. A child with motor and sensory problems should be referred to an occupational therapist.

A referral to CAMHS may be required if the child develops other mental health problems such as Depression or develops obsessions that are impairing.

Many children with ASD attend mainstream schools and may need psychological support from the National Educational Psychological Service in school. They may never need to attend a CAMHS team unless they have a specific mental health problem.

Treatment

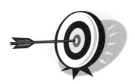

Education & Support
Parents need a lot of support and information to help them understand the symptoms of Autistic Spectrum Disorders and how their child is affected. This will help them understand why a child needs certain types of routine and will explain why many present with unusual behaviours. Such information is vital in working with schools to ensure that the school they choose is the most appropriate for the child.

Behaviour Programme
There are many different behaviour programmes. One such programme is 'The Treatment and Education of Autistic and Related Communication-Handicapped Children' (TEACCH). The focus is on the development of appropriate communication skills and personal behaviours by behavioural training or promoting relationships and self-expression. There is a major emphasis on the way a child with Autism perceives and responds to the environment and to other people. Parents are closely involved in planning the programme and there is an emphasis on visual information with pictures used to help children learn and communicate.

Picture Exchange Programme: PECS
If the child's difficulties are predominantly with communication 'The Picture Exchange Programme' (PECS) can be helpful. PECS uses pictures to help the child express needs and children can exchange a picture of the desired item for the actual item. PECS can also be used to explain what is expected by using a daily timetable. If the child with ASD has adequate language, augmenting teaching with visual aids and instructions can be very helpful.

Social Skills Training

The basic principle of social skills training is to maximise a child's strengths and address areas of difficulty. Appropriate behaviour needs to be explained very clearly and it is essential to ensure the information has been understood. The child then must be encouraged to change difficult behaviour in a stepwise fashion by gradually making small changes. There is a particular focus on the child's positive behaviour and often a reward system can be used to encourage the child.

The 'rules' of social interaction which are intuitive to many children are extremely complex and misunderstood by children with ASD. These 'rules' need to be explained and made personally meaningful to the child and then broken down into small steps to support behaviour change. Praise should be used liberally. If the skills are to be generalised to different settings it is essential that they are practiced across a variety of settings in the child's life, particularly at school and in the home.

Children can be encouraged to use eye contact when communicating. If a child finds eye contact too difficult, he or she can be encouraged to look at another part of the person's face such as the nose or mouth. Some children do not realise that looking at the ceiling or away from the person who is talking can be perceived as rude or inattentive.

Theory of mind – 'Mindreading' CD

This is a computerised game, which is very useful for older children who can read. It consists of different levels of games and puzzles focusing on improving social skills and communication. It teaches children skills for recognising emotions and matching different tones of voice or facial gestures with different emotions.

Medication

Anticonvulsants may be required for seizure control (25 -30% of children with ASD have epilepsy). Stimulants such as Methylphenidate may decrease hyperactivity if the child is very overactive and impulsive. Low dose neuroleptics such as Risperidone may decrease problem behaviours, however, the consequences of long-term use are not known.

Myths

Children with Autism never make eye contact.

Many children with Autism make eye contact but often it is less than normal. It can be just a quick glance or it can be intense, as some children may stare for long periods at a person's face.

Children with Autism cannot show affection.

Sometimes children with Autism may appear aloof and may have difficulty understanding the feelings of others. Also, children with Autism process sensory information differently and may not like hugs or physical contact. It is essential to understand such difficulties and allow the child to express affection without forcing physical contact. Some children with ASD develop close and empathic relationships with more familiar care-givers such as parents and teachers. The most important thing is to find some way of making a connection with the child.

Resources

Organizations

The July Education Programme. This is a funding arrangement for schools to provide further special needs education in the month of July. Special schools and mainstream primary schools with special classes catering for children with Autism may extend their education services for the month of July. If schools are not participating in the July Programme, home tuition is offered as an alternative.

Asperger Syndrome Association of Ireland, Main office, Carmichael House, North Brunswick Street, Dublin 7.

Tel: 01-8780027

Fax 01-8735283   www.aspire-irl.org

The Irish Society for Autism.

asperger@email.com

The Irish Society for Autism, Unity Building, 16/17 Lower O' Connell
Street, Dublin 1. Tel: 01-8744684. Fax: 01-8744224. Educational provision
and support for persons with Autistic Spectrum Disorders.

The Report of the Task Force on Autism, October 2001, Department of
Education and Science.

An Evaluation of Educational Provision for Children with Autistic Spectrum Disorders
-A report by the Inspectorate of the Department of Education and Science,
2006

Books

Asperger Syndrome: A Guide for Parents and Professionals, by Tony Attwood. Jessica
Kingsley Publishers, 1998.

*What does it mean to be me? A Workbook explaining Self Awareness and Life Lessons to the
Child or Youth with High Functioning Autism or Asperger's.* Faherty, C. (2000). Future
horizons, Inc., 721 W. Abraham Street, Arlington, Texas 76013.

How to write Social Stories. Gray, C. (1993a), Future horizons, Inc., 721 W.
Abraham Street, Arlington, Texas 76013.

Writing Social Stories. Gray, C. (2000), Accompanying Workbook to Video. Future
horizons, Inc., 721 W. Abraham Street, Arlington, Texas 76013.

The Curious Incident of the Dog in the Night-time by Mark Haddon. Jonathan Cape,
2003.

Teaching Children with Autism to Mind- Read: A Practical Guide. Patricia Howlin,
Simon Baron-Cohen, Julie Hadwin.

Chapter 4 Autistic Spectrum Disorders

I am Special. Introducing Children and Young People to their Autistic Spectrum Disorder. Vermeulen, P. (2000). Jessica Kingsley Publishers Ltd., 116 Pentonville Road, London N1 9 JB. England.

Why does Chris do that? By Tony Atwood. The National Autistic Society, 1993, website: htpp://www.nas.org.uk

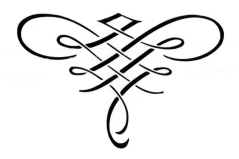

5 Conduct Disorder

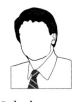

John's story

John is a 14 year old boy who was suspended from school for deliberately lighting a fire in the school yard. His parents are separated and he has witnessed domestic violence at home. He spends very little time at home and regularly stays out all night. His friends are mainly older teenagers who are frequently in trouble with the police for shoplifting and joyriding. He is aggressive towards his peers and his teachers and finds it difficult to obey the school rules...

What is Conduct Disorder?

Conduct Disorder is a serious behavioural and emotional disorder that can occur in children and adolescents. The criteria include a spectrum of unacceptable behaviour from running away from home, stealing from parents to robbery, rape and arson. The central feature of Conduct Disorder is the violation of the rights of others and the disregard for age - appropriate social norms of behaviour.

The *DSM IV* diagnosis of Conduct Disorder is based on the following characteristic symptoms

A repetitive and persistent pattern of behaviour in which the basic rights of others or major age-appropriate societal norms or rules are violated, as manifested by the presence of three (or more) of the following criteria in the past 12 months, with at least one criterion present in the previous 6 months.

- Aggression to people and animals
   often bullies, threatens, or intimidates others
   often initiates physical fights
   has used a weapon that can cause serious physical harm to others (e.g. a bat, brick, broken bottle, knife, gun)
   has been physically cruel to people
   has been physically cruel to animals
   has stolen while confronting a victim (e.g. mugging, purse snatching, extortion, armed robbery)
   has forced someone into sexual activity

- Destruction of property
   has deliberately engaged in fire setting with the intention of causing serious damage
   has deliberately destroyed others' property (other than by fire setting)

- Deceitfulness or theft
   has broken into someone else's house, building or car

- Often lies to obtain goods or favours or to avoid obligations (i.e. "cons"others)
   has stolen items of nontrivial value without confronting a victim (e.g. shoplifting, but without breaking and entering; forgery)

- Serious violations of rules
   often stays out at night despite parental prohibitions, beginning before age 13 years. Has run away from home overnight at least twice while living in parental or parental surrogate home (or once without returning home for a lengthy period) is often truant from school, beginning before age 13 years

- The disturbance in behaviour causes clinically significant impairment in social, academic, or occupational functioning.

If the individual is age 18 years or older, criteria are not met for Antisocial Personality Disorder.

Reprinted with permission from The Diagnostic and Statistical Manual of Mental Disorders, Text Revision, Fourth Edition, (Copyright 2000). American Psychiatric Association.

How is Conduct Disorder diagnosed?

In order for a child to be diagnosed with Conduct Disorder, there must be a long history (more than six months) of persistent socially unacceptable behaviour which greatly exceeds oppositional traits or 'boldness'. Typical behaviour includes: persistent failure to control behaviour appropriately within socially defined rules and repetitive and persistent pattern of defiance, aggressiveness and anti-social behaviour.

Conduct Disorder is characterised as socialised or unsocialised. Socialised Conduct Disorder is the term used when the young person can integrate well in a peer group. Young people with unsocialized Conduct Disorder do not effectively integrate with a peer group.

What signs should teachers look for?

> Persistent failure to control behaviour appropriately within socially defined rules;
> Destructive behaviour involving destruction of property such as deliberate arson and vandalism;
> Use of a weapon that could seriously harm another person;
> Aggressive behaviour towards others, intimidating others;
> Cruelty to animals;
> Telling lies, shop lifting, mugging;
> Persistently breaking school rules;
> Breaking the law;
> Running away from home overnight and staying out all night without parental permission.

What are the effects of Conduct Disorder?

Young people with Conduct Disorder have no regard for authority or the rights of others. Such antisocial behaviour has serious consequences for society and young people can quickly get into trouble with the law. The young person suffers because there may be a co-existing mental health difficulty which has not been diagnosed. The symptoms of Conduct Disorder can mask other emotional difficulties such as Depression and it is very important if a child has a Conduct Disorder that co-occurring ADHD is excluded as ADHD is very treatable. Lacking the social skills to interact, young people with conduct problems tend to have aggressive tendencies with adults and peers. Children with CD often do not pay attention to social cues and may misinterpret other children as being hostile and react aggressively towards them.

Is it a serious condition?

Conduct Disorder is one of the most frequently occurring mental disorders. It is four times more common in boys than in girls occurring in 6-16% of boys and 2-9% of girls. Approximately 40% of young people with Conduct Disorder become juvenile delinquents. The younger a child develops a Conduct Disorder the more serious the outcome and the more likely that the disorder will persist into adulthood. In the Isle of Wight Study, (Rutter et al, 1970), 3,500 children aged between nine and eleven were assessed to determine if they had physical or mental health difficulties. They were followed up again at the age of 14-15 and 35% of the 93 children who met criteria for Conduct Disorder at 10-11 continued to meet criteria at 14-15 years of age.

Difficult peer relationships are a risk factor for serious Conduct Disorder. Having Conduct Disorder impairs a person's ability to form both personal and professional relationships. Children with CD can be very defiant towards authority figures including parents and teachers. These children may often project a very tough image but often have very low self-esteem. Conduct Disorder is linked with higher rates of crime, poor parenting and social problems. Generally, males with CD have lower income and higher rates of unemployment than males without Conduct Disorder. Girls with late onset Conduct Disorder are at an increased risk of substance abuse, unwanted pregnancies and sexually transmitted diseases.

 ## What causes Conduct Disorder?

Genetic Factors

Research has shown that both genes and environment are involved in the aetiology of Conduct Disorders. Conduct Disorders cluster in families, however, twin studies suggest environmental factors are more important than genetic make-up. It is understood, nonetheless, that certain genes can influence temperament. Research has demonstrated an association with these genes, environmental factors and the rate of criminality.

Psychological Factors

Research has shown that if children are maltreated and not brought up in a structured, caring environment with some appropriate limits on behaviour, the risk of developing Conduct Disorder increases. If parents use inconsistent, erratic parenting styles or if they themselves have psychological problems and poor parenting skills, this may reinforce negative behaviour.

Family Factors

There is often family discord and parental criminality in families where children develop Conduct Disorder. A number of characteristics of parents of conduct disordered children have been described. They are usually less effective in terminating deviant behaviour, are vague in their instructions to the child, and issue large numbers of commands at the same time. They use more punishment, less praise and set few rules. Family difficulties such as parental conflict, unemployment, poor housing and health problems often exist.

Cultural Factors

The prevalence of Conduct Disorder is highest in deprived inner cities. This is a common finding amongst different cultures. A number of studies have found an association between poverty and CD indicating that this is an important risk factor. However, the specific mechanism by which cultural and social factors lead to the development of conduct problems is not clear. Conduct Disorder is best conceptualised as developing in the context of personality factors which are shaped by interactions with parents and peers and influenced by sociocultural factors.

Will they grow out of it?

Long term prognosis is strongly related to the severity of deviant behaviour. The age of onset of symptoms also has significant prognostic implications. Indeed two factors that best predict outcome are the age when treatment is commenced and severity of symptoms. In conflict situations, children tend to have episodes of intense anger and resort to aggressive actions rather than verbally mediated responses. In such situations, blame is often attributed to peers (for example, "He made me hit him") and children with Conduct Disorder seldom take responsibility for their own actions. If children with CD do not receive any therapeutic intervention and behaviour patterns become ingrained, successful resolution of symptoms is rare.

Conduct Disorder can be a precursor to adult Anti-Social Personality Disorder. Fifty per cent of children with Conduct Disorder go on to develop Anti-Social Personality Disorder. Unfortunately there are few effective interventions. Multisystemic Therapy (MST) is an intensive family and community-based treatment that addresses the externalising behaviour of young people displaying emotional and behavioural disturbances of a serious anti-social kind. To date, MST has been shown to be the most effective treatment of Conduct Disorder.

What can teachers do to help?

In school, clear rules are required and all positive behaviour should be reinforced. A reward system can help children modify behaviour. Teachers can help the child by establishing realistic expectations in which the child is likely to succeed. It is very important to praise the child for any positive behaviour, especially pro-social behaviour.

It is important to try to help children with low self-esteem. Most children with CD have very low self-esteem and they may have internalised negative feelings about self-worth. As well as a child's own experiences, development of self-esteem is dependent on parental attitudes, experiences and opinions. It is also affected by other significant people in the child's life, including teachers and peers.

The child will require significant support to learn social skills from peers. The class teacher is well placed to model appropriate social behaviour. It is very important that the child gets clear and consistent feedback and understands what is acceptable behaviour in school and what is not. Putting limits on unwanted behaviour in a firm but supportive way will help the child to learn how to behave in different situations. Immediate feedback is very important to prevent situations escalating to a crisis.

Another strategy that may be useful is "time out". This method is a means of extracting the child from an unproductive interaction and consists of placing the child in a quiet space for a period so that no attention is given to him or her and negative behaviour is not inadvertently reinforced with attention. If time out strategies are being used, it is important that the child understands how long time out is for. Otherwise it can invoke feelings of abandonment or rejection from peers.

Peers can be a great help for modelling social skills and this can be done in a fun way using team work and pairs. A model of cooperation rather than competition can be encouraged. Children who are aggressive often misinterpret situations in their environment and attribute hostile intent to others in ambiguous situations. They often select action oriented solutions to their problems rather than reflective solutions. The more help the child can get in reading social situations correctly and learning problem solving skills, the less outbursts and misunderstandings that should occur.

It is very important that one member of staff tries to build a positive relationship with the child. Children are more motivated to improve behaviour if they like and respect their teacher. Good school-home communication can be very helpful as parents may sabotage school rules and policies if they do not understand or are unaware of them. It is also crucial to attend to any learning or reading difficulties that the child may have.

When is professional help needed?

Professional help is needed when children are out of control in the classroom setting and when they will not conform to the usual strategies used for behaviour management. A low threshold for referral to services may significantly limit the child developing long term problems.

Treatment

Many approaches can be taken:

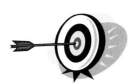

➤ Multisystemic Therapy (MST) services are delivered in the home, school and community. The treatment plan is designed in collaboration with the young person, family and all relevant agencies working with the child. It is a very practical and goal-orientated treatment. It targets the behaviours that are problematic for the child and also provides the child with a support network;

➤ Parent training is the treatment of choice for conduct problems in children under ten years old, particularly those with moderately severe symptoms, less coexisting problems and less social disadvantage;

➤ Sometimes individual self-esteem work can hugely boost confidence as children may have been subjected to harsh criticism and rejection in the past;

➤ It is very important to remember that often these young people may have undiagnosed ADHD or Depression and it is essential that this is diagnosed and managed;

➤ For older children (8-12 years) with more severe presentations, parent training should be combined with individual interventions that provide problem solving and social skills training;

➤ Target additional problems such as substance abuse, academic failure and poor peer group support;

➤ Medication may have a role in severely aggressive behaviour, especially if present with other mental health problems. However, this would always be part of a multimodal treatment response;

➤ Consistent parenting with limit setting and clear boundaries are required without using very punitive or coercive methods.

Myths

Troubled adolescents just need more discipline.
Almost 20% of youths in trouble with the law have a serious emotional disturbance and of this 20% most have a diagnosable mental disorder.

Resources

The Incredible Years: A Trouble Shooting Guide for Parents of Children aged 3 to 8. Webster Stratton C., 1992. *London: Umbrella Press.*

Bringing up responsible Children. Sharry, J. 1999. Veritas.

Bringing up responsible Teenagers. Sharry, J. 2001. Veritas.

Chapter 5 Conduct Disorder

Psychosocial disturbances in Young People, Challenges for Prevention. Rutter, M.,
   Cambridge: Cambridge University Press

Antisocial Behaviour by Young People. Cambridge: Cambridge University Press.
   Rutter, M., Gilder, H., Haggle, A. 1988

Actions speaks louder: A handbook of nonverbal Group Techniques, 1999, 6th edition,
   Revoker, PJ., et Scorch, ET, Churchill Livingstone

Games for social and Life Skills, 1986, Bond, T. Nelson Thomas

Reference

Rutter, M., Tizard, J., Whitmore, K: *Education, Health and Behaviour: Biological and
   Medical Study of Child Development.* London, Longman Group Ltd.

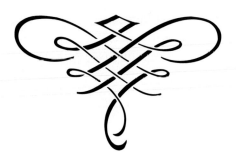

6 Developmental Coordination Disorder

David's story

David is an 8 year-old boy who can not tie his shoelaces and often puts his clothes on back-to-front. He has difficulty using a knife and fork and prefers to use a spoon or to eat with his hands. He is very clumsy and often bumps into things or knocks things over. At school he is fidgety in his chair and has trouble keeping his attention on tasks. He has poor writing skills…

What is Developmental Coordination Disorder?

Developmental Coordination Disorder (DCD) is a term used to describe delayed development of motor skills resulting in poor coordination and clumsiness. Children with DCD lack the coordination required to carry out everyday tasks appropriate for their age and intelligence. Early identification and intervention is very important. There are often associated learning, speech and language and attention problems. Children with intellectual disability or ADHD may also have DCD.

DSM IV Criteria for Developmental Coordination Disorder

> **A**. Performance in daily activities that require motor coordination is substantially below that expected given the person's chronological age and measured intelligence. This may be manifested by marked delays in achieving motor milestones (e.g., walking, crawling, sitting), dropping things, "clumsiness," poor performance in sports, or poor handwriting.
> **B**. The disturbance in Criterion A significantly interferes with academic achievement or activities of daily living

Reprinted with permission from The Diagnostic and Statistical Manual of Mental Disorders, Text Revision, Fourth Edition, (Copyright 2000). American Psychiatric Association.

How is Developmental Coordination Disorder diagnosed?

The diagnosis is based on the criteria outlined above, however, in order to be diagnosed with DCD there cannot be another neurological disorder which could account for the motor difficulties. To meet the criteria for diagnosis, the child's movement problems can not be due to any other known physical, neurological or behavioural disorders.

What signs should I look for?

> Poor handwriting skills;
> Difficulty using a knife and fork;
> Clumsiness in sport;
> Difficulty tying laces and doing zips;

➢ Speech and language difficulties;

➢ Frequent bumping into things and knocking things over

➢ Reduced attention and concentration;

➢ Difficulty tuning out non-relevant stimuli in the environment.

What are the effects of Developmental Coordination Disorder?

Children with difficulties with motor control often appear clumsy. The reason for this is because the child may have proprioceptive difficulties and not know where their limbs are in space. This may cause the child to lean too hard on their pencil and break it or not lean hard enough to write or draw properly. The child may have a lot of difficulties with activities that require constant changes of body posture or adaptation to changes in surroundings such as P.E. and certain sports. Children may become uninterested in sporting activities and for boys in particular this can significantly reduce social contact with peers.

The child may have difficulty with visual motor coordination which is how most motor tasks are coordinated. The consequence of this is that the child may have difficulty with very basic tasks such as dressing, using a knife and fork or for example using building blocks. Children may have difficulty reading due to poor eye coordination which can lead to blurred vision and the child may consequently skip lines of text.

Children with DCD often have difficulty processing the information they receive from their senses. These include: smell, touch, hearing, sight, taste and movement. Figure-ground discrimination is the ability to select and focus on one object despite being surrounded by numerous stimuli. These stimuli can be visual or auditory. If the child is unable to focus on one stimulus at a time, it can result in the child being overwhelmed with multiple sources of information at the same time. This in turn affects a child's ability to read or pay attention.

Every child with DCD may be affected differently, however if certain areas of difficulty are targeted significant improvements can be seen. Children with DCD can become very frustrated and this may result in low self-esteem as the child may perceive motor difficulties as the result of being "stupid or lazy". Early diagnosis can help improve skills, educational performance and social competencies which will in turn enhance self-esteem.

Can anyone develop Developmental Coordination?

Research has shown that DCD is present in 6% of children between the ages of five and twelve. It tends to occur more frequently in boys.

Is Developmental Coordination Disorder a new phenomenon?

Since the early twentieth century there have been reports of children with movement skill difficulties. Over the years it has been called "clumsy child syndrome", "physically awkward children" and Dyspraxia. Dyspraxia is a specific difficulty in motor planning and is actually a subtype of DCD. DCD is a syndrome which was recognised by the World Health Organization in 1992 and has been in diagnostic manuals since 1989.

 ## What causes Developmental Coordination Disorder?

DCD arises when there is a difficulty in the processing of information between the brain and the body. There is no one cause of DCD and it is considered to be a neurodevelopmental disorder resulting from an immaturity in the developing brain. Children with DCD have perceptual difficulties as a result of motor coordination, proprioception and sensory integration difficulties. The sensory system detects pressure, light, taste, smell and texture. All information is interpreted from the environment through receptors and brought to the brain cortex for processing.

It is thought that the brain's ability to process information in DCD may be the result of inadequate connections between the nerve cells in the brain. Proprioception is awareness of body position. Muscle receptors react to the degree of contraction or relaxation within the muscle and transmit signals to the brain as to where each limb is. This system is dysregulated in DCD and if for example, a child with DCD wishes to place a cup on the table, the relevant signals are not picked up and transmitted resulting in difficulty with working out how far to stretch to reach the table and how much force to apply in putting the cup down. This can result in the child accidentally banging the table with the cup.

Genetic Factors

To date there are no genetic markers that can reliably identify the disorder.

Family Factors

There is some evidence that DCD occurs in children where there is a family history of specific learning difficulties.

Cultural Factors

DCD occurs across all cultures and ethnic groups.

What can the teacher do to help?

In the classroom it is important to identify the areas in which a child has specific difficulties.

➤ The child may benefit from sitting near the front of the classroom as less distractions are likely and the teacher is in a position to redirect;

➤ It can be helpful to break tasks down into small steps and wait until the child masters each one before introducing new concepts;

➤ Frequent repetition may be needed to learn new skills and the child may require a lot of support and prompting;

➤ The child should be allowed to take breaks when tired as it may take a lot longer to complete tasks compared to peers;

➤ Use mime games and play word games with children to help increase knowledge and improve memory skills;

➤ Encourage some sporting activity and sequences of movements such as throwing and catching a ball when stationary, then throwing and catching when moving;

➤ Help the child to be aware of the positions of the body in space, for example, at desk, in line, when talking to teachers or peers.

➤ Ensure that the child is positioned properly at the desk, sitting at the midline of the desk with feet touching the floor. A cushion may be necessary;

➤ The child's writing material should be in a similar position;

➤ Handwriting can be difficult for a number of reasons including poor posture, poor fine motor skills which affects pen grip, difficulties with motor planning to coordinate all the skills needed to write;

➢ The child should stabilise paper with one hand while writing;

➢ Some children find that thicker pencils and grips are easier to hold. If the child finds it hard to balance the page on the desk, perhaps it could be taped onto the desk;

➢ Often children will start writing a line in the middle of the page or will start at the left and slope downwards diagonally. Lined paper can be very helpful. It is also helpful to put a marker or star on the left hand side of the page so the child remembers where to begin and a mark on the right hand side to remind the child to go horizontally across the page;

➢ If handwriting becomes a significant issue even after intervention, consider allowing the child to use a computer or writing aid;

➢ If the child has difficulties with letter formation, draw the letter on the palm of the child's hand with a finger. Ask the child to visualise as well as feel the shape of the letter. Sandpaper stencils can be used to allow the child to feel the shape of the letter. This kinaesthetic approach increases the likelihood that handwriting will improve.

When is professional help needed?

If the child's difficulties are affecting everyday life at home and in school, professional help is required. Some children have significant difficulties with tasks such as getting dressed and toilet training. If this is the case, an assessment with a full multidisciplinary team is recommended. If a child is not presenting with any emotional difficulties, referral to CAMHS is not required; in this case management by a speech and language therapist or occupational therapist in the community is preferable.

Treatment

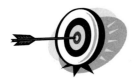

➢ The child needs a medical assessment to rule out all potential physical causes including cerebral palsy, muscular dystrophy or global developmental delay;

➢ Education about Developmental Coordination Disorder is very important for parents and teachers working with the child;

➢ The child needs to be helped to develop an awareness of individual strengths as well as limitations to allow the child to adapt and manage everyday tasks and to promote self-esteem;
➢ An individual plan needs to be made for each child;
➢ The child may need assessment by an occupational therapist to address fine and gross motor skills and may benefit from Sensory Integration Therapy;
➢ Speech and Language Therapy may be required to address any specific speech and language difficulties.

Myths

Children with DCD are just lazy.
DCD is a term used to describe difficulties in the development of motor skills and associated learning, speech and language and attention problems. Children often have to try harder than peers to succeed. However, repetitive failure may lead to low self-esteem and poor effort which may be perceived as laziness. Continuing praise and empathy will help.

They will grow out of it.
The condition affects a child's performance of everyday tasks and children tend not to "grow out of it". The reality is that many adults with DCD struggle to carry out normal everyday tasks.

Resources

Cocks, N. 1996, *Watch me, I can do it! Helping children overcome clumsy and uncoordinated motor skills.* Sydney: Simon & Schuster.

Culligan, B. 2009, *Spelling and Handwriting*. A Guide for Teachers and Parents.

Report of the Task Force on Dyslexia, July 2001, Department of Education and Science.

Understanding Dyslexia. A DVD / CD -Rom for parents and teachers of children with Dyslexia, June 2005. Department of Education and Science.

Sweeney, C., *Good Inclusive Practice for Children with Dyspraxia/DCD in Irish Primary Schools*. Dyspraxia Association of Ireland.

Dyspraxia Association of Ireland,
c/o 389 Ryevale Lawns, Leixlip, Co. Kildare. tel: 0035312957125

National Learning Network, Head Office, Rosyln Park, Beach Road, Sandymount, Dublin 4,
Tel: 0035312057344
Fax: 0035312057376

7 Eating Disorders

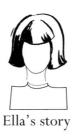

Ella's story

Ella is fourteen years old. She first started to become conscious of her weight when she was preparing for a school play in first year. She started a diet at that time, which has increasingly spiralled out of control. She now restricts herself to eating only fruit and tiny pieces of bread crusts. She has dropped three stone and is significantly underweight. However, she does not accept that this is the case, believing that she is "fat". She exercises repetitively when given any chance. When in class she constantly moves her feet under the table to burn calories. Her schoolwork has significantly deteriorated. She lacks concentration and is increasingly isolated from peers...

What is Anorexia Nervosa?

Anorexia Nervosa is one particular type of Eating Disorder which negatively affects the person's relationship with food and body image. It causes the young person to become preoccupied with weight and body shape to the point that weight loss becomes a central feature of life. Thoughts about body shape and about food become distorted by illness and consequently the person has difficulty making any realistic appraisals about food intake or the individual's own body shape. Behaviour becomes almost solely directed towards the goal of weight loss with previous interests becoming secondary and relationships with friends and family frequently becoming strained as others struggle to comprehend the behaviour.

Distinguishing 'normal dieting' from Eating Disorder Symptoms

- Denial of being "on a diet" despite obvious restriction and weight loss;
- Denial of hunger or craving;
- Claims of needing less food than others;
- Change in food 'rules', e.g. vegetarianism, not eating after 6pm;
- Attempts to hide weight loss, e.g. wearing baggy clothes;
- Increased interest in food/cooking for others;
- Unusual eating behaviours: eating very slowly, chopping food up into tiny amounts, segregating foods;
- Eating alone;
- Bathroom trips after eating;
- Ritualised behaviours;
- Social isolation, low mood;
- Increased exercise.

How is Anorexia Nervosa diagnosed?

The **DSM-IV** diagnosis of Anorexia Nervosa is based on the following characteristic symptoms.

- Refusal to maintain body weight at or above a minimally normal weight for age and height (e.g., weight loss leading to maintenance of body weight less than 85% of that expected; or failure to make expected weight gain during period of growth, leading to body weight less than 85% of that expected).
- Intense fear of gaining weight or becoming fat, even though underweight.
- Disturbance in the way in which one's body weight or shape is experienced, undue influence of body shape on self-evaluation, or denial of the seriousness of the current low body weight.
- In postmenarcheal females, amenorrhoea, i.e., the absence of at least three consecutive menstrual cycles.

Reprinted with permission from The Diagnostic and Statistical Manual of Mental Disorders, Text Revision, Fourth Edition, (Copyright 2000). American Psychiatric Association.

What signs should I look out for?

- ➢ Noticeable weight loss;
- ➢ Avoidance of eating with others;
- ➢ School lunches left unfinished or thrown away;
- ➢ When eating, moving food around the plate repetitively or cutting food into very small pieces;
- ➢ Using bathroom immediately after eating;
- ➢ Excessive exercise, fidgeting, running, skipping;
- ➢ Frequent excuses to explain not eating;
- ➢ Minimisation of weight loss.

What are the effects of Anorexia?

- ➢ Low mood;
- ➢ Low energy;
- ➢ Decreased concentration;

➢ Decreased ability to perform to potential in exams and work environment;

➢ Loss of confidence;

➢ Loss of enjoyment of activities;

➢ Increasing social isolation and avoidance of friends.

Physical Complications:

Cardiovascular: Low blood pressure and heart rate. Changes and abnormalities in heart rhythm. The child may complain of feeling weak, dizzy or faint.

Gastrointestinal: Slow stomach emptying, bloating, decreased motility in the gastrointestinal system. These may all lead to a feeling of fullness even after eating only a very small amount. There may also be high cholesterol, and abnormal liver function tests.

Renal: Dehydration, kidney stones, abnormal kidney function tests, passing urine more frequently and ankle swelling.

Haematological: Anaemia. Iron deficiency.

Endocrine: Abnormal thyroid functioning, growth failure, osteopenia, swollen salivary glands and amenorrhoea.

Menstrual cycle disturbance and potential infertility.

Central Nervous System: thinning of the brain, seizures.

Other: Dry scaly skin,
　　　　Muscle wasting and "lanugo" hair (fine downy type hair) on the face;
　　　　Increased risk of osteoporosis;
　　　　Cold extremities;
　　　　Weakness and fainting.

Is it a serious condition?

Anorexia is a potentially life-threatening condition, particularly if it is left for a long time without being treated. There is a high mortality rate (approximately 5% per decade) both from medical complications and from suicide. Progress in treatment is frequently slow. Approximately 50% recover and one third have chronic symptoms. The earlier treatment is initiated the better.

Can anyone develop Anorexia Nervosa?

Approximately one in a hundred people have Anorexia Nervosa. It is about 10 times more common in girls than boys. The most common time to develop Anorexia Nervosa is late adolescence (70% present between age 12 and 24) but even primary school children may be affected. 10% of eating disorders present before the age of 11 and under age 12 the female to male ratio is 4:1.

Is Anorexia Nervosa a 'new phenomenon'?

Anorexia Nervosa has been described since the 1860s. Despite concerns about media representation of a very thin body ideal, studies have not demonstrated a true increase in the prevalence of Anorexia Nervosa. More people with Anorexia, however, are now being recognised and seeking treatment, which may have contributed to the incorrect assumption that prevalence has increased.

Until recently, there were no figures available on the numbers of Irish teenagers with eating disorders. Consequently, a large-scale study, *Eating Problems in Children and Adolescents*, EPICA, (McNicholas) took place across 52 schools in Ireland and 3,138 teenagers were screened for the presence of eating disorder symptoms. From this data, it was found that nearly 11% of the girls had significant eating concerns and 1.2% of girls were identified as being 'at risk' of Anorexia Nervosa. This study found that in general those with pathological eating concerns were more overweight, exercised less when compared to peers who did not have eating concerns and used dieting and vomiting as a means to monitor weight. They were also more likely to be dissatisfied with quality of life, friends and academic performance and were more depressed than those not preoccupied with weight and shape. They were also more likely to be adversely affected by the media portrayal of ideal weight and shape.

What Causes Anorexia Nervosa?

There is no single cause of Anorexia Nervosa and it is described as 'multifactorial' in origin. The young person may be predisposed to developing the illness for a number of reasons including individual factors, family factors and cultural factors. Anorexia Nervosa may develop following a 'normal' diet which goes out of control. The 'trigger' for Anorexia could be one or more of a multiplicity of factors. For example, in a young person who is vulnerable to developing an Eating Disorder, the trigger could be a stressful life-event such as an exam or bereavement or critical comment by a peer about shape and size. The young person may experience the control of food intake as helping to minimise the effects of other stresses.

Genetic Factors

Researchers have proven that Anorexia Nervosa has a genetic component. This has been explored by research with identical twins. It has been shown that when one identical twin has Anorexia Nervosa, the other twin is more likely to develop the illness when compared to non-identical twins. This provides proof of the genetic contribution to the development of Anorexia Nervosa, as the greater the genetic similarity the higher the likelihood of developing the illness. There is also an increased rate of Eating Disorder in siblings. Furthermore, parents who themselves have eating concerns may pass this on to children.

Psychological Factors

There are a number of psychological theories that have been proposed to explain the development of Anorexia Nervosa. People who develop Anorexia Nervosa are commonly noted to have perfectionistic traits. A person with Anorexia Nervosa typically bases self-worth on thinness. Some theorists have suggested that Anorexia Nervosa develops as a result of the young person's fear of growing up. This theory proposes that the young person with Anorexia Nervosa prevents sexual development by not eating and consequently maintaining the body in a prepubertal state.

Familial Factors

The classic description of a family where a child has Anorexia Nervosa is 'enmeshed'. This describes a family that is rigid, avoids overt conflict and is overly protective. While this description may occasionally be valid, it does not invariably apply. Furthermore, it is not fully clear whether this interactional style is the result rather than the cause of having a child with Anorexia Nervosa. What is most important is that clinicians do not 'blame' families for a child developing Anorexia Nervosa, as parents and families are most important in successful treatment.

Cultural Factors

As mentioned above, there has been much recent debate in the popular media about the role of the 'size zero culture' in precipitating Anorexia Nervosa. In the Irish EPICA study the majority of students felt that the media pressure to be thin had a negative effect on their overall quality of life, with more girls being affected than boys. Research has established that Anorexia is more common in certain groups such as ballet dancers and models. Despite anecdotal evidence that Anorexia Nervosa is becoming increasingly prevalent in Ireland, there are no research statistics available to confirm this. However, it is worth noting that there has been an increase in the rates of dieting in all children, especially teenage girls (between 20% and 50% are on a diet). Recent research has shown that 80% of 10-year-old girls in the USA have dieted or are currently on a diet. At the age of 6, 40% of American girls wish they were thinner. Dieting is in turn a risk factor for Anorexia Nervosa.

What can the teacher do to help?

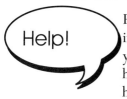

Prevention of the development of Eating Disorders is very important. Given the increasing prevalence of dieting in young people, it is important to support children in healthy weight loss when necessary. Furthermore, obesity has increased at an alarming rate. In Ireland it is now regarded as one of the more prevalent chronic diseases of childhood.

Nutritional information can be provided in SPHE. Attention needs also to be given to increasing children's self-esteem, and to prevent vulnerable children valuing and judging themselves based on weight and shape alone. The student and teacher may find it helpful to have a discussion acknowledging the particular difficulty that the student has with food and agreeing on details of how this will be managed during school-time. It can be worthwhile to be specific in these discussions. For example, agreeing with the student the terms the teacher will use to signify break-time and the length of time that the student will be given to finish lunch.

If it is practicable within the particular school environment, it is helpful to identify with the student's parents, snacks that can be made available to ensure that the student is eating over the course of the school day.

It is helpful if the student can be facilitated to feel more comfortable by eating in a small group setting to avoid feeling overwhelmed in the school canteen.

If possible, the student should be offered some flexibility with regard to snack time. The student may find it easier to eat in situations while engaged in another activity as opposed to at lunchtime when the primary focus is eating.

Flexibility may also be required if the student is becoming upset or distracted from schoolwork due to the presence of food or food odours. In this case it may be helpful to allow the student to complete work in a different class environment.

When is professional help needed?

If a teacher suspects that a student may have an eating disorder, the student's parents should be informed and advised to bring their child to a GP. The GP will then assess the child's medical and psychiatric well-being and make a decision regarding the need to refer to specialist services.

Treatment

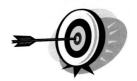

The overall aim of treatment is to:
1) restore a healthy Body Mass Index.
2) change the faulty, maladaptive thinking that is integral to Anorexia Nervosa, for example, morbid fear of fatness, belief that one is fat despite evidence to the contrary.
3) address other non- food/ weight issues such as maturity fears, perfectionism and interpersonal relationship problems.

The general clinical approach is to encourage a stepwise return to a balanced diet using 'behavioural' principles. The person's target Body Mass Index (wt/ht^2) is calculated as is target daily calorific intake (which increases as treatment progresses). A 'contract' is agreed with the young person that details rewards which are contingent on successfully reaching an agreed target. The contract also establishes the consequences for the young person if calorific intake is not maintained. For example, a teenage girl who is being treated as an inpatient, might be 'contracted' to achieving her calorific intake for 3 days if she is to have hours at home with her family at the weekend. Failure to do so will mean she has to forfeit her trip home.

Psychoeducation is a fundamental aspect of treatment. This involves increasing the young person's awareness of the need for regular meals and regular exercise. Providing the family with information on Eating Disorders and the physical, behavioural and psychological effects of starvation is essential.

Cognitive-Behavioural Therapy is also used in the treatment of Anorexia Nevosa. This form of therapy focuses on helping the young person challenge beliefs about thinness, body-shape, food and exercise. The young person is helped to make links between thinking about food and weight and behaviour, such as restricting food intake. The young person is encouraged to see the link between thoughts such as 'I am fat' and feeling states such as sadness and to develop alternative strategies to deal with these thoughts.

It is essential to involve families in the treatment of young people with Anorexia Nervosa. The aim of involving family is firstly to provide information to help understand the disorder. It is very important to help the family to 'externalise' or separate the disorder from the child. This allows the family to express frustration with the disorder without disparaging the child. For example, 'I hate what Anorexia is doing to this family' versus 'I hate you'. Parents are empowered to take charge and to get the child to eat. They also work with the clinician to look at any stressors on the child by exploring family functioning and communication within the family.

DSM–IV Diagnostic Criteria for Bulimia Nervosa

A. Recurrent episodes of binge eating. An episode of binge eating is characterized by both of the following:
- Eating, in a discrete period of time (e.g., within any 2-hour period), an amount of food that is definitely larger than most people would eat during a similar period of time and under similar circumstances.
- A sense of lack of control over eating during the episode (e.g., a feeling that one cannot stop eating or control what or how much one is eating).

B. Recurrent inappropriate compensatory behaviour in order to prevent weight gain, such as self-induced vomiting, misuse of laxatives, diuretics, enemas, or other medications; fasting, or excessive exercise.

C. The binge eating and inappropriate compensatory behaviours occur, on average, at least twice a week for three months.

D. Self-evaluation is unduly influenced by body shape and weight.

F. The disturbance does not occur exclusively during episodes of Anorexia Nervosa.

Type: Purging Type vs. Non-purging Type (exercise & fasting to compensate).

Reprinted with permission from The Diagnostic and Statistical Manual of Mental Disorders, Text Revision, Fourth Edition, (Copyright 2000). American Psychiatric Association.

What signs should I look out for?

➤ Weight loss or unusual fluctuations in weight;
➤ Alternating restricted and binge pattern of eating;
➤ Large amounts of food disappearing from cupboards;
➤ Use of bathroom immediately after meals;
➤ Preoccupation with food.

What are the effects of Bulimia?

Largely similar to Anorexia Nervosa
➤ Low mood;
➤ Low energy;
➤ Decreased concentration;
➤ Decreased ability to perform to potential in exams and work environment;
➤ Loss of confidence;
➤ Loss of enjoyment of activities;
➤ Menstrual cycle disturbance and potential infertility;
➤ Increasing social isolation and avoidance of friends.

The physical effects include:
➤ Increased risk of osteoporosis;
➤ Repeated vomiting can lead to a number of complications. Oesophagitis which is an inflammation of the oesophagus may occur and causes symptoms of heartburn and chest pains. If the vomiting is severe, persistent tears can develop in the wall of the oesophagus leading to bleeding which may be life threatening. Severe vomiting can also result in electrolyte imbalances such as low potassium levels. Electrolyte imbalances can lead to cardiac problems such as abnormal heart rhythms;
➤ Calluses may occur on the back of the hands from rubbing on the teeth to induce vomiting;
➤ Inflammation of the pancreas leading to abdominal pain may occur
➤ The salivary glands can become enlarged and painful;

➢ Acid from the stomach may wear away the enamel of the teeth
  leading to tooth decay and gum disease;

Is it a serious condition?

The overall prognosis for someone with Bulimia is better than for Anorexia
Nervosa. Approximately one third of people with Bulimia will remain
continuously ill. Relapses are extremely common and occur in
approximately 60% of people with Bulimia. Depression very frequently
co-occurs.

Can anyone develop Bulimia Nervosa?

Bulimia Nervosa is more common than Anorexia Nervosa and affects
approximately 1% of female adolescents. About 30% of people with Bulimia
will have had Anorexia Nervosa. Frequently, young people with Bulimia
describe a long history of dietary problems. The peak age of onset tends to be
later than for Anorexia Nervosa, occurring in late adolescence and early
twenties. In the EPICA study of 3,138 Irish students, 1.5% were identified as
being 'at risk' of developing Bulimia Nervosa. Although the global levels of
eating concern among Irish adolescents are comparable to those established
internationally, there is a suggestion that Irish adolescents may demonstrate
higher levels of bulimic type behaviours and concerns.

What causes Bulimia Nervosa?

As with Anorexia Nervosa, the causes of Bulimia are
multi-factorial and similar to those mentioned above.

Biological
Genetic studies have revealed that there is a genetic contribution to Bulimia
Nervosa. Chemical transmitters in the brain such as serotonin and dopamine
have also been studied and have been found to be lower than the levels found
in people without Bulimia.

Psychological
Young people with Bulimia have been found to show high rates of Depression and alcohol misuse. They also commonly describe feelings of impulsivity and low self-esteem. Occasionally, there is a history of sexual abuse.

Familial
Families of young people with Bulimia have been noticed to demonstrate high levels of other mental health difficulties, particularly Depression.

What can teachers do to help?

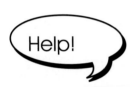

Talk about healthy eating in class discussions. The avoidance of severe, restrictive diets has a direct impact on decreasing bingeing. This in turn decreases the associated feelings of guilt and depression associated with bingeing. Ultimately, preventing restrictive dieting prevents the cycle of dieting, bingeing, guilt and depression leading to more dieting.

If possible, it is very helpful, within the constraints of the school environment, to limit the opportunities that the student has to engage in bulimic behaviour during the school day. For example, allow the student to visit the bathroom prior to eating and ensure that they remain in class for sufficient time (20 minutes) after eating to ensure that food is digested.

When is Professional Help required?

It is best to mention any concerns regarding possible Bulimia to parents and to advise that they bring their child to their GP. The GP will then assess the child for the presence of Bulimia Nervosa as well as checking their physical health.

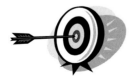

Treatment

As with Anorexia Nervosa, the treatment of Bulimia involves many different therapeutic approaches. Most young people with Bulimia can be treated as outpatients. Helping the young person to understand the importance of healthy eating with a regular diet is a cornerstone of treatment.

Cognitive Behavioural Therapy can be very helpful in enabling the young person to challenge distorted beliefs about food and diet. Overvalued ideas about body shape and weight can be replaced with more realistic and helpful thinking. The young person can be helped to understand more about the emotional cues that trigger bingeing and restricting patterns of eating. This awareness can facilitate changes in the young person's relationship to food by generating alternative, healthier responses to situations that would previously have triggered a binge or purge.

Family work is also important in helping parents to understand their child's difficulties.

Interpersonal Therapy (IPT) may be very helpful in older adolescents where there are often difficulties with relationships.

Medication: Antidepressants such as Fluoxetine can be helpful in the short term both for comorbid depression and reducing binges.

Resources

Useful websites

Bodywhys

PO Box 105, Blackrock, Co.Dublin

Local Helpline: 1890 200 444

Email: info@bodywhys.ie

Website: www.bodywhys.ie

Eating Disorders Association

103 Prince of Wales Road

Norwich

NR1 1DW

UK

Email: info@edauk.com

Website: www.edauk.com. This is the leading UK website for people with eating disorders and their families. Postal address: Beat, 103 Prince of Wales Road, Norwich, NR1 1DW, United Kingdom.

YoungMinds

102-108 Clerkenwell Road,

London EC1M 5SA

UK

Patient's Information Service: (UK) 0800 018 2138

Website: www.youngminds.org.uk

National Institute for Clinical Excellence

Midcity Place,

71 High Holborn

London

WC1V 6NA

Email: nice@nice.hns.ie

Website: www.nice.org.uk

Books

Eating disorders: a parents' guide. Rachel Bryant-Waugh and Bryan Lask (2004). Brunner Routledge.

Breaking free from anorexia nervosa: a survival guide for families, friends and sufferers
Janet Treasure (1987). Psychology Press.

Getting better bit(e) by bit(e): survival kit for sufferers of bulimia nervosa and binge
  eating disorders. Ulrike Schmidt and Janet Treasure (1993). Lawrence Erlbaum

Anorexia nervosa: the wish to change. A.H. Crisp et al (1996). Psychology Press.

Overcoming Binge Eating. Christopher G. Fairburn (1995).Guilford Press.

Bulimia Nervosa: a guide to recovery. Peter J. Cooper (1993). Robinson Publishing.

Anorexia nervosa and related eating disorders in childhood and adolescence 3rd
  edition. Bryan Lask and Rachel Bryant-Waugh (2007). Routledge.

Treatment manual for anorexia nervosa: a family-based approach. James E. Lock
  (2002). Guilford Press
Just take a bite. Lori Ernsperger and Tania Stegen-Hanson (2004). Future Horizons

The following two publications are available from:
Royal College of Psychiatrists Research Unit
  4th Floor Standon House
  21 Mansell Street, London E1 8AA
  Tel: 020 7977 6655
  Web: www.focusproject.org.uk/publications

Eating problems in children: Information for parent(s). Claudine Fox and Carol
  Joughin (2002).

Childhood-onset eating problems: findings from research. Claudine Fox and Carol
  Joughin (2002)

References
McNicholas F, Lydon A, Lennon R, Dooley B (2009) *Eating concerns and media*
  influences in an Irish adolescent context Eur Eat Disord Rev 17(3):203-13

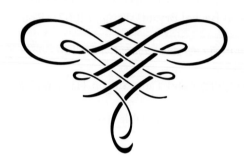

8 Mood Disorders, Depression, Bipolar Affective Disorder

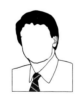

Simon's story

Simon was a 14 year old boy. He had become very quiet and withdrawn in himself over a 3 month period. He used to have lots of friends and play football. Now he preferred to be on his own in his room. When his parents tried to talk to him he was angry and irritable with them. His school work began to decline and he found it difficult to concentrate on his school work. His appetite was reduced and he seemed to be tired and lacking in energy...

What is a Mood Disorder?

Mood Disorder is a term that is applied to a number of conditions in which the most prominent symptom is the depression or elevation of mood.

What is Depression?

Everyone feels sad at times. However, a typical feeling of sadness is transient and does not last more than a few days. If, however, this sad feeling persists and lasts more than two weeks and interferes with everyday life it is likely that the person is depressed.

Most people with Depression experience a number of the following symptoms: feeling unhappy most of the time, loss of interest in life and inability to enjoy simple activities and pastimes, difficulty making decisions, tiredness, agitation, either loss or gain in appetite and weight, change in sleep, early morning wakening, sleeplessness and irritability. In fact many children and teenagers who are depressed are often noticed by parents to be irritable as opposed to sad.

School-age children who are depressed find it hard to concentrate and may lose interest in work and play. Some may even refuse to go to school while others complain of feeling lonely even when they have friends. Some children become irritable and difficult to manage while others lose confidence. Younger children may often develop a lot of physical symptoms.

How is Depression diagnosed?

The DSM–IV diagnosis of Major Depressive disorder is based on the following characteristic symptoms:

Five (or more) of the following symptoms have been present during the same 2-week period and represent a change from previous functioning; at least one of the symptoms is either (1) depressed mood or (2) loss of interest or pleasure.

Note: Do not include symptoms that are clearly due to a general medical condition, or mood-incongruent delusions or hallucinations.

- (1) depressed mood most of the day, nearly every day, as indicated by either subjective report (e.g., feels sad or empty) or observation made by others (e.g., appears tearful).
  Note: In children and adolescents, can be irritable mood
- (2) markedly diminished interest or pleasure in all, or almost all, activities most of the day, nearly every day (as indicated by either subjective account or observation made by others)
- (3) significant weight loss when not dieting or weight gain (e.g., a change of more than 5% body weight in a month), or decrease or increase in appetite nearly every day.
- Note: In children, consider failure to make expected weight gains.
- (4) insomnia or hypersomnia nearly every day
- (5) psychomotor agitation or retardation nearly every day (observable by others, not merely subjective feelings of restlessness or being slowed down)
- (6) fatigue or loss of energy nearly every day
- (7) feelings of worthlessness or excessive or inappropriate guilt (which may be delusional) nearly every day (not merely self reproach or guilt about being sick)
- (8) diminished ability to think or concentrate, or indecisiveness, nearly every day (either by subjective account or as observed by others)

Reprinted with permission from The Diagnostic and Statistical Manual of Mental Disorders, Text Revision, Fourth Edition, (Copyright 2000). American Psychiatric Association.

What signs should teachers look for?

> A change in the child's normal behaviour, mood or academic functioning;
> Extreme moodiness and lack of communication;

➢ Dropping out of hobbies, groups and clubs;

➢ Underperforming at school;

➢ Finding it hard to concentrate, becoming withdrawn and losing touch with friends;

➢ Poor self-care;

➢ Not eating enough or eating too much;

➢ Being very self-critical;

➢ Sleeping badly or sleeping too much or being excessively tired in school;

➢ Physically slowed down;

➢ Feelings of helplessness and worthlessness;

➢ Overreaction to criticism;

➢ Thoughts about suicide or about not wanting to be in this world anymore.

What are the effects of Depression?

➢ The child's mood may be very low or irritable;

➢ Irritability can lead to conflict with peers, teachers and family;

➢ The child may frequently complain of physical symptoms such as headaches and stomach pain;

➢ Children's thought processes can be slowed down and reasoning can be distorted;

➢ Children can become preoccupied with sad, worrying and distressing thoughts and can have difficulty making decisions;

➢ Sleep can be very disturbed, leading to low energy and further impair concentration;

➢ The child may experience a sense of hopelessness and lose enthusiasm and capacity for enjoyment;

➢ Being depressed limits the child's learning, interaction with peers and while depressed the child is at risk of self-harm;

➢ Adolescents may escape from these feelings by drinking, taking drugs or getting into dangerous situations;

➢ If a person becomes very depressed, preoccupation with death and suicide attempts are common.

Is it a serious condition?

If Depression is untreated it can last for months and can impair a young person's functioning at home, with peers and in school. Depressed young people are more likely to attempt suicide. Depression can also exacerbate medical illness. Most children with Depression will get over symptoms in time even without treatment, however for many Depression recurs. Therefore, despite natural remissions it is important to identify Depression as soon as possible and to treat it. For many children, Depression may return and represent a chronic disorder. It is very important to identify such children and to ensure that the illness is adequately treated.

Can anyone develop Depression?

Major depressive disorder affects 2% of children and is twice as common as diabetes. It becomes more common with increasing age. Between 5-10% of adolescents will have a major depressive episode during their adolescent years. In childhood, boys and girls are equally affected but in adolescence it is three times more common in girls.

Is Depression a new phenomenon?

There have been many descriptions of Depression in history. For example, King Saul is described in the Old Testament as experiencing Depression and ended his life by suicide. Depression was first described by Abraham in 1911 and was further developed by Freud in 1917 in a paper called 'Mourning and Melancholia' in which he drew attention to the similarities between mourning and Depression.

What causes Depression?

Like most mental health disorders, the cause of Depression is not completely understood but the evidence suggests it is a combination of genetic and environmental factors and sometimes early adverse experiences. Depressive disorders in young people may be triggered by stressful life events such as bullying, abuse or parental separation. These are usually precipitants for Depression in a person who is already predisposed to becoming depressed. Much depends on the context for the young person, its meaning for the young person and what happens after the event.

Genetic Factors

Depression can run in families which implies that it is inherited. If either parent has depression, the children are 8 times more likely to become depressed than in families where neither parent is depressed. Research has shown rates for identical twins as 45-50% and 25% for non-identical twins. This indicates that although genetic factors are important other factors play a significant role in causing Depression.

Psychological Factors

Depression can be caused by repeated losses or repeated trauma. If a young person is exposed to repeated trauma which appears to have no escape, the child may ultimately feel hopeless. This may lead to a phenomenon described as 'learned helplessness' which in essence describes a person who has learned that attempting to make things better is futile and therefore has given up. This is thought to be the pathway to Depression in some.

Familial Factors

Family influences can be significant when the child may feel unloved or unwanted. Often high expressed emotion - for example, negative, critical, hostile comments can have a profound effect on a child's self-esteem and coping skills. Children are psychologically vulnerable to any conflict in the environment around them. Negative family interactions and conflict have been shown to contribute to children developing Depression.

Cultural Factors

In Ireland women complain of depressive symptoms more often than men. Men are more likely to complain of physical symptoms or try to self-medicate with alcohol when they are feeling depressed. This pattern is seen in many other cultures too.

What can the teacher do to help?

Children with depression may find it very difficult to concentrate in school and may require a reduced workload for a short time. There should be strategies in the school to address stressful situations such as bullying and additional stressors such as exams, especially in vulnerable children.

Suicidal thoughts or self-harm behaviour should be taken very seriously. It is critical that parents are informed and advised to discuss the situation with a GP.

Children who are depressed can find it difficult to find the motivation to plan and should be included in planning activities as much as possible. Children who are reluctant to engage in activities should be gently encouraged to do so.

It is often very helpful to be available to listen to the child's worries. Children with depression need to be praised when they have done something well as often depression results in low self-esteem and the young person's negative thinking may preclude them from recognising things they are managing to do well. Frequently, reminding children of their successes and achievements, whilst helping them cope with adversity or failure is important.

When is professional help needed?

If a child is thought to have Depression, an assessment should be arranged to clarify the diagnosis. If a child has been underperforming in school, has lost interest in peers and expresses thoughts that life is not worth living, clinical assessment is required.

Treatment

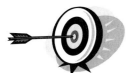

The child needs to be seen by a medical doctor to rule out any physical cause for these symptoms, such as Anaemia (low iron levels).

The majority of children with depression should be referred to the local CAMHS team. Most children are treated as outpatients. If children require more intensive input, however, either due to the severity of their depressive thoughts, the risk of self-harm or adverse family situations, they may require either a day hospital or inpatient admission.

Attending a Child and Adolescent Mental Health (CAMH) team

A full assessment is carried out to confirm the diagnosis of Depression. It is essential as part of the assessment to identify child and family strengths and supports. Information is provided about Depression. Potential stressors in the child's environment are explored and if any immediate stress is identified which is modifiable, parents are advised to act.

Cognitive Behaviour Therapy

CBT helps the young person to identify and monitor states of negative feeling, replace negative thoughts with more balanced thoughts and to incorporate an increasing range of healthy behaviour (regular sleep, exercise, socialising, hobbies) in weekly schedules. CBT aims to improve a young person's mood through developing an understanding of how thoughts, feelings and behaviour are linked.

A child who is depressed often fears the worst (I'll never pass my exams), is self-critical (I'm never any good at anything) and only sees the bad side of things (I only passed my mocks because they marked the papers too easily).

CBT works by helping to restructure a child's thoughts, perceptions and beliefs which can facilitate emotional and behavioural change. It helps the child adopt a more positive and balanced view on things; for example, 'this is a hard exam but I usually pass' or 'although I am struggling with maths, I find many other subjects easy'.

Family Therapy

Parenting a child with depression is very challenging for a variety of reasons. It can be extremely difficult for parents to see their child so obviously sad and withdrawn. Parents may experience guilt and blame themselves for their child's difficulties. Sometimes parents can experience a sense of helplessness or anger with the child for not 'just getting better'.

During family therapy, relationships, roles and communication styles are explored in detail. Family therapy can help families to improve their relationships with each other and also help families to identify unhelpful family dynamics that lead to increased tension and stress at home. It aims to stop unhelpful interactions amongst family members, help the family to communicate better and improve relationships. This will help parents support their child and respond to the child's needs. The identification and treatment of depression in parents is also important.

Antidepressant Medications

Antidepressants work by altering neurotransmitters in the brain. Neurotransmitters are chemicals which transmit signals between cells in the brain. In depression, two neurotransmitters, serotonin and noradrenaline, do not seem to work properly. Antidepressants work by increasing the activity and availability of these chemicals in the brain.

Antidepressants are used to treat moderate to severe depression. They take approximately 2-3 weeks to work, however some people report a small improvement in their symptoms after 2-3 days.

All antidepressant medications have side-effects, which are carefully discussed with the child and parents before starting the medication. The most common side-effects are nausea and vomiting. Medication, if used, is always only one aspect of a treatment plan and needs to be carefully monitored.

Myths

Adolescents do not suffer from "real" depressive illnesses — they are just moody.
Adolescents can frequently (5-10%) suffer depressive episodes and it is very important that this is recognized early and that they receive appropriate support and help.

Depression only happens when something bad happens.

Depression can be triggered by things going wrong, for example, break up of a relationship. However it can also occur for no apparent reason and this is due to a chemical imbalance in the brain.

Depression is just a form of weakness.
Depression is an illness and can affect anyone.

Bipolar Affective Disorder

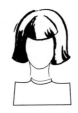

Caroline's story

Caroline is a 15 year old girl in her Junior Certificate year. She started becoming irritable at home and in school and everyone thought that she was "just stressed". She began to stay up all night and seemed to have abundant energy. She became very talkative and started shouting out inappropriate comments in class which was unusual for her as she was previously very shy. When answering a question in school she seemed to be easily distractible and not follow her sentences through but jump from one topic to another. She became exhausted from her lack of sleep but seemed to be unable to slow down and relax. She began to boast that she was famous and was going to leave school as she had been chosen to join a major new girl band....

What is Bipolar Affective Disorder?

Bipolar Affective Disorder is a serious but treatable disorder manifested by severe mood swings from 'lows' to 'highs'. The periods of highs and lows are called episodes of mania and depression both of which can result in serious impairment of a person's functioning. These shifts in mood are markedly more extreme than normal ups and downs. The symptoms include marked

106

changes in mood, energy, thinking and behaviour. Mania is defined as a persistent state of extreme elation or irritability with grandiose ideas accompanied by high energy. In some people, symptoms of mania and Depression can occur at the same time. This is called a mixed bipolar state.

How is Bipolar Affective Disorder diagnosed?

The DSM- IV diagnosis of Bipolar Affective Disorder is based on the following characteristic symptoms.

Manic episode

- A distinct period of abnormally and persistently elevated, expansive, or irritable mood, lasting at least 1 week (or any duration if hospitalization is necessary).
- During the period of mood disturbance, three (or more) of the following symptoms have persisted (four if the mood is only irritable) and have been present to a significant degree:
    - inflated self-esteem or grandiosity;
    - decreased need for sleep (e.g., feels rested after only 3 hours of sleep);
    - more talkative than usual or pressure to keep talking;
    - flight of ideas or subjective experience that thoughts are racing;
    - distractibility (i.e., attention too easily drawn to unimportant or irrelevant external stimuli);
    - increase in goal directed activity (either socially, at work or school, or sexually) or psychomotor agitation;
    - excessive involvement in pleasurable activities that have a high potential for painful consequences (e.g., engaging in unrestrained buying sprees, sexual indiscretions, or foolish business investments).

Reprinted with permission from The Diagnostic and Statistical Manual of Mental Disorders, Text Revision, Fourth Edition, (Copyright 2000). American Psychiatric Association.

What signs should teachers look for?

 Manic children are more likely to present with irritability, whereas older adolescents and adults present with elated mood and grandiosity. Children may appear disorganised, giddy and have difficulty concentrating. If there is a marked deterioration in a child's performance with associated moody behaviour, it is important to have the child assessed.

What are the effects of Bipolar Affective Disorder?

There can be increased speed in thought processes with consequent increased rate of speech. The young person's conversation may jump from one unconnected topic to another. Children can have a decreased need for sleep. When a young person is in a manic phase of illness, judgement can be seriously impaired and may result in extremely risky behaviour. Children may be irritable, distractible and have trouble concentrating. This can lead to very significant interference with a child's school work as well as relationships with friends and teachers.

Young people with untreated Bipolar Affective Disorder can experience manic episodes lasting about three months and depressive episodes can last over a year. It affects a person's family, school and social life. During a manic phase there is a higher risk of unplanned, teenage pregnancy and young people can become very disinhibited in their behaviour, commit crimes and end up in trouble with the law. People with the disorder may also develop alcohol or drug related problems.

Can anyone develop Bipolar Affective Disorder?

Bipolar Disorder occurs in approximately 1 in 200 children and tends to run in families. Recent studies of adults with bipolar illness show that many had their first episode of bipolar illness before age 17.

Is Bipolar Affective Disorder a new phenomenon?

It has been recognised since at least the time of Hippocrates who described such patients as "amic" and "melancholic". In 1899 Emil Kraepelin defined manic–depressive illness. In 1921 Kraeplin observed that mania was rarely observed in children and that onsets of first episode increased after puberty. Nowadays it is increasingly recognised in younger children, particularly in the United States . It is more difficult to diagnose in young children who may frequently have very short mood swings which last only a few hours. The child may have highs and lows many times in the same day.

What causes Bipolar Affective Disorder?

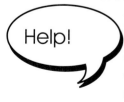 It is thought to be caused by a number of contributing factors, including genetic, biochemical and environmental. A number of neurotransmitters have been linked to this disorder including serotonin and noradrenaline

Genetic

For people with Bipolar Affective Disorder there is risk of Depression or Bipolar Disorder in 1 out of 5 of first degree relatives. Rates of 60–70% for identical twins and 20% for non-identical twins have been cited. When one parent has Bipolar Disorder the risk to each child is 15–30%. If both parents have Bipolar Disorder the risk increases to 50–75%.

Familial

In addition Bipolar Affective Disorder runs in families in part due to a genetic risk. Stress in the family can make a relapse more likely. It is important that families learn to recognise triggers and do their best to reduce levels of negative expressed emotion in the home.

Cultural

Men and women are equally affected by Bipolar Disorder. It is more commonly diagnosed in the USA where children who are irritable, hyperactive and disorganised can be diagnosed as having Bipolar Affective Disorder. Providing regular follow up and review assessments will help avoid misdiagnosis.

What can teachers do to help?

Help! Firstly, it is important to discuss your concerns with the student's parents to gain a comprehensive understanding of the young person's difficulties. It is crucial to be mindful of the child's difficulties when providing sanctions and consequences to misbehaviour. It is important to avoid overstimulation and allow time out if necessary.

Teachers can look for any triggers in the school setting which may make a student's mood worse. It may be useful for the teacher to keep a note of changes in the young person's behaviour and to discuss with the student on an individual basis possible precipitants or stressors in the school environment which are contributing to mood/behaviour changes. When the teacher and student have developed a clear and shared understanding of stressors, it is then possible for the teacher to problem-solve with the young person to minimise the impact of the potential stressors and maximise the student's capacity to cope. The child may need help to organise themselves in class and may have difficulties with short-term memory.

Often young people with Bipolar Disorder do not realise when they are unwell and may have unrealistic goals. They may need help to plan their school timetable which may need to be altered at certain times when the young person is unwell.

When is professional help needed?

Professional help is required when the young person is so disorganised that there is evidence of objective impairment and functional decline. If the young person is engaging in serious risk-taking behaviour or expressing suicidal ideation an urgent referral to the local CAMHS team is required.

Treatment

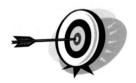

The child needs to be seen by a medical doctor to rule out any physical cause for mood symptoms and a range of blood tests will be checked. The child usually needs referral to the local CAMHS team. The initial treatment plan will include education about the symptoms of Bipolar Affective Disorder. Bipolar Affective Disorder needs to be treated with medication as well as other therapies.

Cognitive Behavioural Therapy

In therapy the young person is encouraged to recognise any triggers that affect mood and to become aware of mood changes by keeping a 'mood diary'. CBT helps people with Bipolar Disorder to learn to become more in control of the emotional response evoked by particular thought patterns. CBT seeks to enable the young person to minimise the impact of the illness by regularising daily routines (exercise and sleep) and learning to recognise early signs of relapse (the individual's relapse signature). It is important that young people and their families can learn to recognise signs of relapse so that early intervention can be sought before a full blown episode occurs.

Family Therapy

The focus of family therapy is on communication skills and problem-solving skills. In therapy, family members are supported to look at their healthy and unhealthy responses to problems that arise in the family system.

Families get the chance to explore problem-solving skills, effective communication skills and manage their child's symptomatic behaviour. It is important that the home environment is supportive and that stressful situations are quickly diffused and managed by parents.

If a parent has symptoms suggestive of a mood disorder it is important that the appropriate treatment is received. A depressed parent is less able to support and respond to the child's needs .

Medication

Mood stabilisers act to stabilise the young person's mood. They can be very effective in controlling mania and preventing the recurrence of both manic and depressive episodes. Several types of mood stabilisers are available including Lithium, Carbamazepine and Valproate. Other medications are added when necessary for shorter periods to treat episodes of depression or mania that are not managed by a mood stabiliser alone. Bipolar Disorder is a recurrent illness, so long term medication is usually indicated.

Myths

People with manic depression are dangerously unstable and generally drop out of society.
Manic depression– or Bipolar Disorder– is a serious mental illness, which may cause significant distress and affect personal relationships. However many people with Bipolar Disorder lead full and meaningful lives. In fact some of the most brilliant creative individuals are thought to have suffered from Bipolar Disorder including many statesmen, actors and comedians.

When people are manic with Bipolar Affective Disorder they are very happy.

Many people are very irritable and unhappy when they become manic. Lack of sleep and disorganisation leads to increasing distress.

People with Bipolar Affective Disorder never recover.

Many people make a full recovery with effective treatment.

Bipolar Affective Disorder only affects mood.

Bipolar Affective disorder affects judgement, memory, energy, appetite, sleep and self-esteem.

Resources

Aware – Helping to defeat Depression, Helpline Tel: 1890303302. Postal address: 72 Lower Leeson Street, Dublin 2. Email: wecanhelp@aware.ie

Responding to Critical Incidents. Guidelines for Schools. National Educational Psychological Service, Department of Education and Science (2008).

Responding to Critical Incidents. Resource Material for Schools. National Educational Psychological Service, Department of Education and Science (2008).

Reach Out: National Strategy for Action on Suicide Prevention (2005). Health Service Executive National Suicide Review Group. Department of Health and Children.

Useful websites

National Institute of Mental Health (NIMH), Office of communications and public Liaison, Information resources and Inquiries, 6001 Executive Blvd., Rm. 8184, MSC 9663, Bethesda, MD 20892–9663,
phone: (301) 443–4513, Fax: (301) 443–4279
Email: nimhinfo@nih.gov, website: www.nimh.nih.gov
Changing Minds: Mental Health: What is it, What to do, Where to go? A multimedia CD–ROM on mental health that looks at depression. www.changingminds.co.uk

Child & Adolescent Bipolar Foundation, 1187 Wilmette Avenue, PMB # 331, Wilmette, IL 60091, Phone; (847) 256–8525

Chapter 8 Bipolar Affective Disorder

www.bpkids.org
www.bipolarworld.net

www.youngminds.org.uk

Books

Young Minds provides information and advice on child mental health issues102–108, Clerkenwell Road, London EC1M 5SA. Parent's information service 08000182138.

Long, R. 1999, *Understanding and supporting depressed children and young people*. Tamworth: Nasen.

Survival Strategies for parenting children with Bipolar Disorder
Lynn, G. 2000, Jessica Kingsley Publishers, ISBN 1853029211

The Bipolar Disorder Survival Guide: What You and Your Family Need to Know, Milkowitz, D., George, E., 2007, Guildford Press, ISBN 1593853181

The Bipolar Child: The Definitive and Reassuring Guide to Childhood's most misunderstood Disorder, Papolos, D., Papolos, J., 2006, Broadway Books

Deliberate Self Harm in Adolescence, Fox and Hawton (2000)

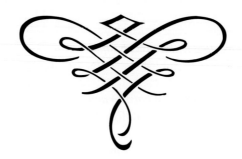

9 Tic Disorders and Tourette Syndrome

John's story

John is a 10 year old boy who developed a repetitive jerking movement of his head and began to make repetitive humming and grunting noises. He disrupted other children in the class as his humming noises became louder when he was anxious. He was teased by other children for this. This went on for over a year and his parents brought him for professional help and a diagnosis of Tourette's Syndrome was made...

What is Tic Disorder?

A tic is an involuntary, rapid, repeated twitch that produces a quick movement that is of sudden onset and serves no apparent purpose. A vocal tic is a sound made involuntarily. Vocal tics may be as innocuous as humming, throat clearing, clicking or more obvious such as barking and grunting. Complex vocal tics include repetition of certain words and sometimes the use of unacceptable or obscene words. This is known as coprolalia. Tics may involve different parts of the body. The most common motor tics are eye-blinking, nose twitching, shrugging of shoulders and facial grimacing. Complex motor tics include hitting oneself, jumping, touching parts of one's own body, pelvic thrusting or whole body jerking.

The nature and complexity of tics varies over time. The natural course of tics is to decrease in intensity for periods of time (weeks to months) and then recur. They usually subside when the child is engrossed in an activity and stop when the child is asleep. Transient tics are very common, especially in boys, starting at around the age of 7 or 8. If tics last a long time (more than 1 year), it is known as a Chronic Motor Disorder. Less frequently, a child may present with vocal tics only.

The DSM–IV diagnosis of Tic Disorder is based on the following characteristic symptoms

- Chronic Motor or Vocal Tic Disorder;
- Single or multiple motor or vocal tics (i.e., sudden, rapid, recurrent, nonrhythmic, stereotyped motor movements or vocalizations), but not both, have been present at some time during the illness;
- The tics occur many times a day nearly every day or intermittently throughout a period of more than 1 year, and during this period there was never a tic-free period of more than 3 consecutive months;
- The onset is before age 18 years;
- The disturbance is not due to the direct physiological effects of a substance (e.g., stimulants) or a general medical condition (e.g., Huntington's disease or postviral encephalitis).
- Criteria have never been met for Tourette's Syndrome

Reprinted with permission from The Diagnostic and Statistical Manual of Mental Disorders, Text Revision, Fourth Edition, (Copyright 2000). American Psychiatric Association.

The DSM–IV diagnosis of Tourette's Syndrome is based on the following characteristic symptoms

- Both multiple motor and one or more vocal tics have been present at some time during the illness, although not necessarily concurrently. (A tic is a sudden, rapid, recurrent, non-rhythmic, stereotyped motor movement or vocalization).
- The tics occur many times a day (usually in bouts) nearly every day or intermittently throughout a period of more than 1 year, and during this period there was never a tic-free period of more than three consecutive months.
- The onset is before age 18 years.
- The disturbance is not due to the direct physiological effects of a substance (e.g., stimulants) or a general medical condition (e.g., Huntington's Disease or Postviral Encephalitis).

Reprinted with permission from The Diagnostic and Statistical Manual of Mental Disorders, Text Revision, Fourth Edition, (Copyright 2000). American Psychiatric Association.

What is Tourette's Syndrome?

A child with Tourette Syndrome has **both** motor and vocal tics present for more than one year. Tourette's Syndrome is a lifelong condition but in many cases tics become less obvious as people get older.

What signs should I look for?

The signs can vary as tics can come and go and change in frequency over time. The child may be disruptive in class and may pretend that the tics were voluntary in order to cover up embarrassment. Motor tics commonly present as blinking, grimacing and nose-twitching. Common vocal tics include tongue clicking, voice clearing and grunting.

What are the effects of Tic Disorder?

The effects vary depending on the severity of the child's tics. If a child has mild tics they tend not to cause too much disruption. However, if they are complex and frequently occurring they can affect a child's ability to concentrate, sit still, hold a pen and write and may lead to bullying or ridicule from peers. 40% of children with Tourette Syndrome have attention problems. Tics can have a major influence on a young person's confidence and self-esteem.

Is it a serious condition?

In some cases tics can be voluntarily suppressed and hardly noticeable. In others, the tics can be severe and interfere with all aspects of a child's life. Tourette's Syndrome is usually a life-long disorder although periods of remission can occur. Tic Disorder usually improves during adolescence and symptoms usually diminish entirely by early adulthood. Tic disorders tend to be exacerbated by stressful life events, however some children's tics worsen when they are bored or fatigued.

Can anyone develop Tics?

Transient Tic Disorder is common in the early school years. It affects 5% to 24% of all children. It differs from Tourette's Syndrome in that the tics occur daily for at least two weeks but for no longer than one year. Chronic Tic Disorder is when there are either vocal or motor tics that last for more than one year. Tourette's Syndrome occurs in four per 1,000 of the population. It is three times more common in males than females.

Are Tics a new phenomenon?

Tourette's Syndrome is also known as Gilles de la Tourette Syndrome after the neurologist who described the disorder in 1885. In 1825, the first description of a patient with Tourette's Syndrome appeared in a paper by Itard who described a woman who displayed not only involuntary tics but also obscene vocalisations.

What causes Tic Disorder and Tourette's Syndrome?

Tourette Syndrome is inherited genetically and transient tic disorders are more common in first degree relatives than in the general population. Both twin and family studies have shown that genetic factors are implicated in the transmission of Tourette's Syndrome and related tic disorders. At present it is thought that many genes may be involved and further research is needed to determine exactly which genes will predispose individuals to develop the disorder. Almost all cases of Tourette's Syndrome result from a combination of genetic and environmental factors. However it can be caused by head trauma, carbon monoxide poisoning and certain viral infections. There is evidence that chemicals in the brain including dopamine, norepinephrine and serotonin are involved.

Genetic Factors

Evidence from twin and family studies suggests that Tourette's Syndrome is an inherited disorder. Recent family studies show that the pattern of inheritance is complex and involves more than one gene. Genetic predisposition may not necessarily result in full blown Tourette's Syndrome, instead it may be expressed as a mild tic disorder. As the inheritance pattern is unclear it is difficult to determine who may be at risk of developing the condition.

At least 50% of children with Tourette's Syndrome develop obsessive compulsive symptoms by adulthood and 60% of children with OCD have a history of tics ranging from mild tics to Tourette's. Studies have shown that 50-70% of children with Tourette's Syndrome also have ADHD. Researchers have linked Tourette's to an area of the brain called the basal ganglia. This structure is deep in the brain and relays messages between the prefrontal cortex and the lower structures. The basal ganglia is involved in controlling movement and plays an important role in attention, concentration, movement and decision making.

Cultural Factors

Tourette's Syndrome can occur in children of all racial and ethnic backgrounds.

What can the teacher do to help?

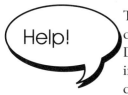

Tic Disorder and Tourette's Syndrome can occur in children of all ability levels. Most children with Tic Disorder and Tourette's Syndrome have normal intelligence. Children with tics or Tourette's Syndrome cannot control these involuntary sounds and movements and should not be blamed for them. The best approach for transient tics is to ignore them as much as possible. A culture of acceptance of strengths and weaknesses amongst the entire class is helpful.

Sometimes the child can suppress the tics voluntarily but this usually builds up and the child then has a series of tics which is sometimes known as a 'tic storm'. If it is not possible to perform these in class, time out of class may be required. If unable to control tics, the child should be allowed to go to a less stimulating area if necessary in order to be less disruptive and not observable by other children.

It can be helpful to allow the child to engage in tic behaviours if necessary at lunch break to relieve anxiety. Attending to these tics in the classroom can distract the child.

Complex tics may result in the child being unable to write or hold a pen so alternative teaching methods may be used, usually visual and auditory aids and perhaps a dictaphone in the classroom. Children with tics are often teased by peers and bullying should be anticipated . Given that tics are frequently associated with both ADHD and OCD, it is important to be on the look out for these symptoms also.

When is professional help needed?

If a child's tics are significantly impacting on everyday functioning, referral to the local GP should be discussed with the parents of the child. The GP can then review the child and determine whether referral to a specialist service is warranted. The disorder can have a negative impact on a child's self-esteem and, if tic behaviours are disruptive, may lead to rejection by peers. If this occurs it is important to bring this to the attention of parents and consider seeking extra help for the child.

Treatment

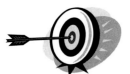

The initial treatment includes support and education about the disorder for child and parents. Anxiety management and relaxation therapy are very useful. CBT and medication are sometimes also needed.

Cognitive Behavioural Therapy

CBT helps children to become aware of the links between thoughts, feelings, behaviours and how they relate to tics. This is known as awareness training.

120

In some cases the child can be helped to recognise the build up to tics ('premonitory urges' and associated thoughts). Many individuals with these urges describe feeling a body sensation such as an urge to clear their throat. These urges, and the internal drive to control them, can create a lot of tension and stress that can only be relieved by performing the tic. If a certain visual or auditory cue precedes a tic then there is an opportunity to intervene and allow the person to learn to identify when situations arise which may worsen tics.

Habit reversal is a strategy used to reduce tics. It works to increase awareness of behaviour and to provide relief with strategies that replace the unwanted behaviour with a less troublesome one. Early detection can be learned and situations which affect frequency of tics can be recognised. The child may learn to engage in competing behaviours such as deliberately moving the head to the right if the tic movement is to the left or sitting on hands to prevent jerking. Children may learn how to mask vocal tics with a cough.

Medication
Sometimes certain medications are used in low doses to reduce complex tics. Examples are Clonidine or a neuroleptic such as Risperidone. If the child has ADHD this may also require treatment.

Family Therapy
It is important to help families develop strategies to help them manage tics. Often parents can help by recognising and reducing any stressful triggers at home that may exacerbate the child's tics. Sometimes it may be easier to suppress tics while at other times individuals report that it may be nearly impossible to suppress them. It is important that parents understand this, as some parents find it frightening that children can manage tics.

Myths

People with Tourette Syndrome can voluntarily suppress tics if they want to.
Tics are caused by a chemical imbalance in the brain. Physical and vocal tics are completely involuntary (much like a sneeze). Although tics can be held back for a short time, after a while they usually need to be released. This can put the individual under considerable tension and lead to stress. The child usually needs to be allowed to engage in the tic behaviour to relieve tension.

All people with Tourette Syndrome swear and use bad language.
A minority of people diagnosed with Tourette Syndrome involuntarily swear and use obscene language which is called Coprolalia. Some also make rude gestures. This is called Copropraxia and is relatively rare.

Resources

Guide to the Diagnosis and Treatment of Tourette Syndrome. www.mentalhealth.com

Organizations

Tourette Syndrome Association of Ireland, Carmichael House, North Brunswick Street, Dublin 7. Tel;018725550

Books

Tourette Syndrome: a practical guide for teachers, parents and carers. Carroll, A. & Robertston, M. (2000). London: David Fulton. ISBN: 1853466565

Living with Tourette Syndrome, Shimburg, E. (1995). New York: Simon & Schuster. ISBN:068481160X

Gilles de la Tourette Syndrome. Shapiro, Arthur K. et al (Eds/C1988). New York: Raven Press.

An Educator's Guide to Tourette Syndrome. Bronheim, S (1994). New York: Tourette Syndrome Association, Inc.

Tourette Syndrome: A Practical Guide for Teachers, Parents and Carers. Carroll, A. & Robertson, M. (2000). London: David Fulton.

Tourette Syndrome: The Facts. Robertson, M. & Baron-Cohen, S. (1998) Oxford. Oxford University Press.

Tourette's Syndrome and Tics: Relevance for School and Psychologists. Wodrich, DL: *Journal of School Psychology: 36 (3) 281-294.*

Tics and Tourette Syndrome: A Handbook for Parents and Professionals. Chowdhury, U. (2004). . Jessica Kingsley Publishers.

Living with Tourette Syndrome. Shumberg, E. (1995). Simon & Schuster Publishing Group.

10 Post-Traumatic Stress Disorder (PTSD)

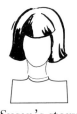

Susan's story

Susan is a 6 year old girl who was involved in a serious car accident. She needed to be cut out of the car and was lying trapped for 30 minutes. She sustained a fractured pelvis and was in hospital for 2 weeks. She began to have repeated nightmares and flashbacks about the accident, reliving the experience on a daily basis. She had interrupted sleep and was tired and stressed. She refused to go into the family car and did not want to go past the road where she had the accident, even though this was the quickest route to school…

What is Post-Traumatic Stress Disorder (PTSD)?

PTSD refers to the development of characteristic symptoms (flashbacks, avoidance and hypervigilance) following exposure to a traumatic event. In the context of PTSD, a traumatic event is defined as an event where a person perceives or witnesses a threat of extreme danger to the individual or someone else. Typical examples are road traffic accidents, assault, rape, being taken hostage, or being diagnosed with a life-threatening illness. Research has shown that it is how a person interprets the situation rather than the actual incident that is significant. Therefore a vast array of different traumas can trigger PTSD. The development of PTSD is also dependent on how an individual processes the trauma. A child may show intense fear, horror, helplessness or agitation. There is often intensification of distress when the child is exposed to reminders of the event and repetitive or intrusive day-dreams or flashbacks. Typical symptoms include episodes of repeated reliving of the trauma, intrusive memories or dreams, a sense of numbness and emotional blunting, avoidance of activities or cues that remind the sufferer of the trauma.

To be diagnosed with PTSD, symptoms must start within 6 months of the traumatic event.

Three main types of symptoms are associated with PTSD:
- Re-experiencing the traumatic event: this is when the person replays the incident over and over again either in play, conversation, thoughts or in dreams.
- Avoidance or emotional numbing: this is when the person avoids the scene where the incident took place, avoids talking about it and seems to shut down feelings.
- Increased arousal: this is when a person seems to be alert, hypervigilant and may be unable to relax.

The DSM–IV diagnosis of Post–traumatic Stress Disorder is based on the following characteristic symptoms

A. The person has been exposed to a traumatic event in which both of the following were present:
- the person experienced, witnessed, or was confronted with an event or events that involved actual or threatened death with serious injury, or a threat to the physical integrity of self or others
- the person's response involved intense fear, helplessness, or horror. Note: In children, this may be expressed instead by disorganized or agitated behaviour

B. The traumatic event is persistently re-experienced in one (or more) of the following ways:
- recurrent and intrusive distressing recollections of the event, including images, thoughts, or perceptions. Note: In young children, repetitive play may occur in which themes or aspects of trauma are expressed
- recurrent distressing dreams of the event. Note: In children, there may be frightening dreams without recognizable content.
- Acting or feeling as if the traumatic event were recurring (includes a sense of reliving the experience, illusions, hallucinations, and dissociative flashback episodes, including those that occur on awakening or when intoxicated).
- Note: In young children, trauma- specific re-enactment may occur.
- intense psychological distress at exposure to internal or external cues that symbolize or resemble an aspect of the traumatic event.
- Physiological reactivity on exposure to internal or external cues that symbolize or resemble an aspect of the traumatic event.

C. Persistent avoidance of stimuli associated with the trauma and numbing of general responsiveness (not present before the trauma), as indicated by three (or more) of the following:
- efforts to avoid thoughts, feelings, or conversations associated with the trauma
- efforts to avoid activities, places or people that arouse recollections of the trauma
- inability to recall an important aspect of the trauma
- markedly diminished interest or participation in significant activities
- feelings of detachment or estrangement from others
- restricted range of affect (e.g., unable to have loving feelings)
- sense of a foreshortened future (e.g., does not expect to have a career, marriage, children, or a normal life span)

D. Persistent symptoms of increased arousal (not present before the trauma), as indicated by two (or more) of the following:
- difficulty falling or staying asleep
- irritability or outbursts of anger
- difficulty concentrating
- hypervigilance
- exaggerated startle response

What signs should teachers look for?

> ➤ Awareness that any child who has experienced a traumatic event may be distressed;
> ➤ Re-enactment of the trauma in spontaneous play or if the child is experiencing flashbacks which are vivid episodes in which the child experiences the trauma as if it were happening again;
> ➤ There may be a change in the child's behaviour, poor performance at schoolwork, lack of interest or irritability;
> ➤ The child may be hypervigilant and have poor concentration; Hypervigilance may present as excessive checking of doors and windows or being very irritable and on edge in school, or jumping when teacher calls name;
> ➤ Children often complain of physical symptoms such as stomach aches and headaches when they are experiencing flashbacks;
> ➤ A reluctance to engage in certain activities (which may be linked to the original traumatic event, e.g. refusal to go on a school outing in a bus).

What are the effects of Post-Traumatic Stress Disorder?

> ➤ The child may attempt to avoid any situation associated with the trauma which may lead to a restricted lifestyle, to separation anxiety and 'clinginess' and a refusal to separate from parents;
> ➤ If parents permit avoidant behaviour, it may prolong the child's recovery time by facilitating ongoing avoidance and thereby not allowing the child to overcome the fear;
> ➤ Avoidance may intensify if the child is forced to face a situation without sufficient preparation;
> ➤ The child may attempt to suppress upsetting feelings ultimately leading to a feeling of numbness;
> ➤ The child may have difficulty falling or staying asleep. Sleep problems are often associated with intense fear of the dark and of

trauma related nightmares. Consequently the child may appear
sleepy or irritable in class;
➢ The impact of unresolved trauma is huge and may affect all aspects of
a child's life.

Is it a serious condition?

Adolescents may resort to drug and alcohol abuse as a way of avoiding the
trauma related effect and dealing with their heightened anxiety. Young
children may lose interest in things that they used to enjoy and they may find
it hard to believe that they will live long enough to grow up. Young people
may also have a foreshortened view of the future, being unable to envisage
growing to maturity and having a long and fulfilling life. This affects their
ability to plan events in the future and often leads young people to make hasty
impulsive decisions without considering the consequences. In general the
more disturbing the experience the more likely a person is to develop PTSD.
It is the individual's perception of the threat to their own safety that is the
most important predictor of PTSD and not the magnitude of the trauma.
PTSD affects the child's beliefs and expectations about the world and their
place in it. PTSD may result in a deeply held but false belief that 'the world is
totally unsafe'. This belief will then have a dramatic influence on the child's
thoughts and behaviour.

Traumatic events undermine the sense that life is fair, reasonably safe and
secure. A traumatic experience makes the vulnerability of life and potential
of dying at any time very clear to the child. This can affect a person's outlook
in life and precipitate feelings of insecurity.

Can anyone develop Post-Traumatic Stress Disorder?

Any individual who experiences a trauma may go on to develop PTSD.
However, it is difficult to predict with accuracy which individuals will suffer
from PTSD after a traumatic event.

3-15% of girls exposed to a trauma and 1-6% of boys who have experienced a
trauma develop PTSD. In adults the lifetime prevalence is 10-12% for
women and 5-6% for men.

Is Post-Traumatic Stress Disorder a new phenomenon?

The first documented case of psychological distress was recorded in 1900 BC by an Egyptian physician who described a "hysterical" reaction to trauma. It was also described in the 19th century when it was called "Hysterical Neurosis". After the First World War, many soldiers developed 'shell shock' as PTSD symptoms were initially attributed to neurological damage, secondary to exploding ammunition shells. PTSD was first introduced as a diagnostic category in 1980. Since this time several studies of children traumatized by various catastrophic situations have appeared.

What causes Post-Traumatic Stress Disorder?

It usually arises as a delayed response to a stressful event or situation of an exceptionally threatening or catastrophic nature which is likely to cause pervasive distress to almost anyone (natural disaster, serious accident, rape, torture, etc.). However, it can also occur with less obvious traumatic experiences if a person perceives it to be an intensely traumatising situation.

Biological Factors
Adrenaline is a hormone produced by stress. In PTSD the vivid memories of trauma keep the levels of adrenaline elevated which may make a person tense or irritable. The hippocampus is a part of the brain that processes memories. High levels of stress hormones can prevent the hippocampus from processing the trauma. When the stress settles, adrenaline levels go back to normal, the disturbing memories can be processed and the flashbacks and nightmares will stop.

Psychological Factors
If a person is extremely frightened, arousal level and perceptions may be increased resulting in a very clear memory of the event. The flashbacks of the event may force the child to think about what has happened and decide what to do if it happens again.

Studies of cognitive processes in children with PTSD arising from exposure to acute stressors have shown that they have memory deficits; they tend to estimate that negative events are more likely to happen to others than to themselves which may be a process of denial. Children who are hypervigilant are on guard waiting for another crisis to happen. This heightened level of arousal facilitates a speedy reaction to potential threats in the environment.

Familial Factors

Family support and parental coping skills have been shown to affect PTSD symptoms in children. If children have good relationships with their parents and families this will provide a secure environment to help them cope if they are exposed to a traumatic incident.

Cultural Factors

Younger children from ethnic minority groups and lower socioeconomic groups may be at increased risk of PTSD. Some studies with adults show that people from Black and Hispanic ethnic groups are more vulnerable to developing PTSD. PTSD is found in elevated rates in refugee children and this is understandable given the multiple episodes of trauma many refugee children have experienced. Many refugees have been traumatised in their own country and often have a very dangerous and difficult journey to seek refuge. Children may be separated from families and this can be compounded by the move to a new country with a different language and culture where the child can feel completely lost.

How can the teacher help?

Help!

The child may be irritable and have angry outbursts leading to difficulties with maintaining peer relationships and conflict with parents and teachers. It is important to be very supportive and understanding towards the child and to help restore a sense of control. Any positive interaction should be praised and a normal routine encouraged where possible. If a child is very anxious or startles easily, it may be useful to encourage relaxation exercises in the classroom.

It may also be helpful to make a plan with the child and the child's parents which recognises that the child may need time out of the class if feeling overwhelmed. A plan is much more likely to be successful if it incorporates specifics such as where the child should go during this time and the exact distraction and calming techniques which should be employed.

When is professional help needed?

When the symptoms of PTSD have led to disruption of a child's ability to develop relationships with peers and learning is negatively impacted, professional help may be needed. Parents should be advised by teachers of any concerns the teacher has and how to access the local CAMHS team or psychological services.

Treatment

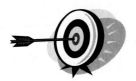

It is important for parents to understand the effects of PTSD on children. Research has shown that in cases where both parents and children have been exposed to the same trauma, the children of parents who manage their own anxiety in the aftermath of the event are less likely to develop PTSD. It is as important for parents to understand the effects of PTSD as it is for children. Research has shown that the better the parents themselves can cope with the trauma, the more they will be able to support the child.

Coping skills are taught to children to help them manage anxiety. This is done by relaxation skills therapy and muscle tension releasing exercises which can be very effective at relieving stress. Children can also learn how to relax when recalling their stressful experiences.

Parent training often includes giving rewards to children for achieving certain goals, such as sleeping in their own bed at night and attending school.

Safety skills training is useful for young people who have been the victims of abuse or violence. Participants are coached to recognise situations where they may not be safe and to have an escape plan ready so that they feel in control.

Individual Approaches

A common approach to managing PTSD is to begin by monitoring the frequency and intensity of symptoms. Firstly, the child is helped to learn anxiety reducing strategies, such as relaxation techniques. A graded exposure to the trauma is facilitated where the child is introduced to the anxiety provoking situation and helped master this before being exposed to a series of increasingly anxiety provoking situations. This needs to be done in a carefully planned way by experienced clinicians.

Cognitive Behavioural Therapy

CBT focuses on the traumatic experiences that have produced the symptoms.

Eye Movement Desensitisation & Reprocessing (EMDR)

Eye Movement Desensitisation & Reprocessing (EMDR) is a technique which uses eye movements to help the brain process flashbacks and to make sense of the traumatic experience. It is combined with CBT and is sometimes used when other therapy has been unsuccessful. During this therapy the patient is asked to visualise flashback and at the same time to be aware of the emotion associated with it. They are then asked to centre this emotion (for example, some people feel it in their stomach) and concentrate on it while they focus their eyes on a moving object in front of them. This process is continued at repeated intervals until the person is able to tolerate the emotions they experience when they have a flashback.

Medication

Sometimes medication is used to reduce the anxiety of the PTSD symptoms and treat any comorbid depression. Again when used it is carefully monitored and part of a treatment plan.

Myths

PTSD only affects war veterans.
Although PTSD does affect war veterans, PTSD can affect anyone exposed to a traumatic event. Victims of trauma related to physical and sexual assault face the greatest risk of developing PTSD.

It is only weak people that can't cope after a traumatic event.
The stress caused by trauma can affect all aspects of a person's life, including mental, emotional and physical well-being. Trauma can affect anyone and most people need a period of readjustment before getting back to their normal lives.

Patients make up symptoms of trauma just to get compensation for PTSD and don't need treatment.

Even though many patients are involved in court cases if they have been involved in accidents, the symptoms of PTSD are very distressing for patients and these patients need treatment even after their court cases are resolved. A delayed court hearing may well complicate treatment.

Resources

Traumatic Stress: The Effects of Overwhelming Experience on Mind, Body, and Society. (1996). Eds. Van der Kolk BA, Mc Farlane AC, & Weisaeth L. Guildford Press. New York, London

Psychological Trauma: *A Developmental Approach.* (1997). Eds. Black D., Newman M., Harris-Hendriks J., & Mezey G. London; Gaskell: The Royal College of Psychiatrists.

Supporting Children with Post-Traumatic Stress Disorder: a practical guide for teachers and processionals (2001). David Kindin and Erico Brown, David Fulton Publishers.

Post Traumatic Stress Disorder: the invisible injury (2005). David Kindin. Success Unlimited.

11 Schizophrenia

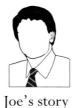

Joe's story

Joe is a sixteen year old boy in Transition year. Joe has always appeared to be slightly on the edge of his peer group. However, recently he seems to be actively avoiding his classmates. On two occasions he has approached teachers with vague allegations that two students had 'sent messages around about him'. When questioned, Joe was unclear as to how this had happened. At times Joe appears completely absorbed by his own thoughts and is very difficult to engage in class work. At other times Joe appears agitated. When Joe does talk, he appears to lose the train of his thought and can be difficult to follow...

What is Schizophrenia?

Schizophrenia is a serious mental illness, which affects many aspects of how a person thinks and perceives the world around them. Schizophrenia can cause people to develop delusional beliefs and hallucinations. Delusions are unshakeable beliefs which are frequently bizarre and which are held with total conviction. Hallucinations occur when a person experiences a sensory stimulus, which they perceive as real but which has not actually occurred. For example, auditory hallucinations occur when the person has the experience of hearing a voice or voices when in fact nobody has spoken. Visual hallucinations occur when the person sees something which is not there in reality. The experience however, is totally 'real' to the person. Schizophrenia also impacts on a person's ability to establish and maintain friendships and to remain in school or employment.

What signs should I look out for?

Increasingly it has been recognised that prior to the onset of a full-blown psychotic episode, the young person has typically been struggling for a considerable period. Furthermore it has been established that the average delay between onset of symptoms and effective treatment is almost 2 years. This places teachers in a very special position of being able to identify early signs and to bring these to the parents' attention. The following symptoms may occur:

- ➤ Significant fall-off in concentration;
- ➤ Deterioration in school-performance;
- ➤ Difficulties getting normal daily activities done;
- ➤ Free-time noticeably less productive;
- ➤ Preference to spending free time alone;
- ➤ Noticeable change in self-care;
- ➤ Noticeable increase in suspiciousness and becoming mistrustful of other people;
- ➤ Taking a particular special and self-referential meaning out of ordinary events;
- ➤ Appearing increasingly absorbed by own thoughts;
- ➤ Appearing increasingly confused by own thinking;

➢ Describing hearing unusual sounds or voices;

➢ Talking about wanting to self-harm or end life;

➢ Talking about harming someone else.

DSM criteria for the diagnosis of Schizophrenia.

A. Characteristic symptoms: Two (or more) of the following, each present for a significant portion of time during a 1-month period (or less if successfully treated):

- (1) delusions
- (2) hallucinations
- (3) disorganized speech (e.g., frequent derailment or incoherence)
- (4) grossly disorganized or catatonic behaviour
- (5) negative symptoms, i.e., affective flattening, alogia, or avolition
- Note: Only one Criterion A symptom is required if delusions are bizarre or hallucinations consist of a voice keeping up a running commentary on the person's behaviour or thoughts, or two or more voices conversing with each other.

B. Social/occupational dysfunction: For a significant portion of the time since the onset of the disturbance, one or more major areas of functioning such as work, interpersonal relations, or self-care are markedly below the level achieved prior to the onset (or when the onset is in childhood or adolescence, failure to achieve expected level of interpersonal, academic, or occupational achievement).

C. Duration: Continuous signs of the disturbance persist for at least 6 months. This 6-month period must include at least 1 month of symptoms (or less if successfully treated) that meet Criterion A (i.e., active-phase symptoms) and may include periods of prodromal or residual symptoms. During these prodromal or residual periods, the signs of the disturbance may be manifested by only negative symptoms or two or more symptoms listed in Criterion A present in an attenuated form (e.g., odd beliefs, unusual perceptual experiences).

D. Schizoaffective and Mood Disorder exclusion: Schizoaffective Disorder and Mood Disorder With Psychotic Features have been ruled out because either (1) no Major Depressive, Manic, or Mixed Episodes have occurred concurrently with the active-phase symptoms; or (2) if mood episodes have occurred during active-phase symptoms, their total duration has been brief relative to the duration of the active and residual periods.

E. Substance/general medical condition exclusion: The disturbance is not due to the direct physiological effects of a substance (e.g., a drug of abuse, a medication) or a general medical condition.

F. Relationship to a Pervasive Developmental Disorder: If there is a history of Autistic Disorder or another Pervasive Developmental Disorder, the additional diagnosis of Schizophrenia is made only if prominent delusions or hallucinations are also present for at least a month (or less if successfully treated).

Reprinted with permission from The Diagnostic and Statistical Manual of Mental Disorders, Text Revision, Fourth Edition, (Copyright 2000). American Psychiatric Association.

Is Schizophrenia a serious condition?

Schizophrenia is a very serious illness that can affect all areas of a young person's life. The earlier Schizophrenia is recognised and treated the better the outcome. A young person who receives early treatment is less likely to require hospital admission and is more likely to go on to live and work independently.

Overall, 20% of people with Schizophrenia will get better within five years of their first episode of illness; 60% will get better but will have relapses and 20% will have persistent symptoms.

Suicide is more common in people with Schizophrenia than in the rest of the population. The period of greatest risk is in the first year after diagnosis. The risk is increased when the person has active psychotic symptoms, has become depressed, is not receiving treatment or when the person has made a previous suicide attempt.

How common is Schizophrenia?

Schizophrenia affects approximately 1% of the population, a prevalence equal to that of diabetes. It is equally common in males and females. It is uncommon to develop Schizophrenia under age 15. The peak incidence occurs between age 15 and 35. Schizophrenia has recently reported to be more common in immigrant populations and in people who have grown up in cities and large towns.

What causes Schizophrenia?

The definite cause of Schizophrenia is unknown. The research to date suggests that it is most likely to be a mixture of different factors such as genetic, biological, social factors and stress. The role that each of these factors plays in the development of the illness for each individual will vary.

Genetic Factors

Genetic factors are known to be important in Schizophrenia. Genes have been shown to account for between 50% to 70% of the risk of developing Schizophrenia. A person with no biological relative with Schizophrenia has a

1 in 100 chance of developing the illness. This risk increases to 1 in 10 for those with one parent with Schizophrenia.

For those with an identical twin with the illness, the risk rises to one in two whereas the risk is considerably lower at one in eighty if the twins are non-identical. Given that identical twins share the exact same genetic make-up, this finding suggests a significant role for genes in the development of Schizophrenia. These differences remain consistent, even in twins that are adopted and reared in different families, adding weight to the theory that it is the genes and not the environment (home life) which makes the significant difference. The genes responsible for Schizophrenia have not been established.

Biological Factors
The neurodevelopmental hypothesis

This theory attempts to link together a number of different research findings on the development of Schizophrenia. It is more common for people with Schizophrenia to have had a viral illness early in their foetal development. It has also been found that babies who experience difficulties at birth resulting in lack of oxygen to the brain have an increased risk of developing Schizophrenia. In addition, brain scans of people with Schizophrenia show that compared to the rest of the population, there are differences in their brains. These studies have established that people with Schizophrenia have higher levels of structural brain abnormalities. Together, these findings suggest a link between damage to the developing brain and development of Schizophrenia in later life.

The use of drugs
The role of specific street-drugs in the development of Schizophrenia has become a topic of increasing interest in recent years.

Research suggests that use of cannabis increases the risk of developing Schizophrenia by 50%. It is important to note that the active drug content in the marijuana which is available today, is very significantly higher than in previous decades. Therefore, it is not possible to draw conclusions as to the long-term mental health effects of cannabis by looking at people that used the drug in past decades. The use of cannabis is more likely to lead to Schizophrenia if the person started using it as a young teenager. The association between cannabis use and development of Schizophrenia is particularly strong for people who have used cannabis more than 50 times: they are 6 times more likely to develop Schizophrenia.

The role of other drugs such as LSD and amphetamines is less clear. For example, it is known that amphetamines can produce transient psychotic states but it is not known if they increase the risk of enduring psychotic symptoms and Schizophrenia.

At times, people who are developing schizophrenia and who have not received any treatment may use drugs and alcohol as a form of self-medication in an attempt to help them deal with distressing symptoms. This may lead to dependence on these substances which makes effective treatment of the illness much more difficult.

Family Factors

Early theories of Schizophrenia emphasised the role of families in its development. Specific styles of communication including a tendency for parents to be inconsistent in the messages they gave their children were thought to be particularly important. It has now been concluded that there is no evidence to support these ideas.

However, it is known that living in an environment where there is expression of high levels of discord (high expressed emotion) within the family leads to a less favourable outcome and increases the likelihood of relapse.

Childhood Deprivation

Children who experience early deprivation or abuse are at increased risk of developing Schizophrenia. Recent research in the Netherlands has demonstrated an increased rate of psychotic illnesses in children who have been abused which has led to increased emphasis on the role of psychosocial factors in the development of these illnesses.

What can teachers do to help?

Early treatment for young people with Schizophrenia is essential. If a teacher notices any of the signs listed above, it is important that concerns are passed on to parents and the young person who should be advised to attend a GP.

When is professional help needed?

Schizophrenia can have very serious negative consequences for young people in all aspects of their life. When concerns arise that a young person may be developing this illness, assessment by a psychiatrist is required as soon as possible. The GP makes an initial assessment of the child and then refers to CAMHS for a comprehensive psychiatric evaluation.

Treatment

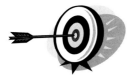 The overall aim of treatment is to reduce psychotic symptoms and to help rehabilitate the person to allow them to reintegrate insofar as is possible to the life led prior to becoming unwell. Treatment may be started in a variety of settings such as in an outpatient department or in hospital depending on how unwell the young person is and taking into account personal and parental views.

When a young person is very unwell with psychotic symptoms, inpatient admission may be required to allow more rapid treatment.

Medication is the cornerstone of treatment in Schizophrenia. The aim is to use medication to decrease the psychotic symptoms over a number of weeks and to help the young person think more clearly again. Ultimately, the goal is to enable the young person to return to as near as possible to their previous level of functioning.

What are the side-effects of medication?

The most commonly prescribed medications for Schizophrenia are called 'atypical' or 'second-generation' anti-psychotics to distinguish them from the original 'first-generation' anti-psychotics that were discovered in the 1950s.

Unfortunately, as with all medication, there are a number of potential side-effects including:
- Drowsiness;
- Increased appetite;
- Weight gain;
- Increased risk of Diabetes;
- Muscle stiffness and shaking in the hands.

Medications are typically started at the lowest possible dose to control symptoms and increased gradually as required to limit the likelihood of side-effects. The young person and parents are made aware of side-effects at the outset. It is important that the young person is aware of the possibility of weight gain. Both the young person and parents are encouraged to pay attention to dietary intake. The need for regular exercise is highlighted as a priority. Blood tests may be taken prior to the start of medication and will be monitored regularly. The effectiveness of the medication in reducing psychotic symptoms is closely assessed. The medication may be increased or switched to a different medication if it does not control symptoms adequately.

How important is medication?

Medication is a core element of treatment. It does not however 'cure' the illness but does play a significant role in helping to keep symptoms at bay. Approximately 80% of people with Schizophrenia who are treated with antipsychotics will experience a reduction in symptoms. Despite this, symptoms may recur even when taking medication. However, the young person is much less likely to have a relapse when taking medication than if medication is stopped prematurely.

Young people are generally advised to take medication for at least one year following a first psychotic episode. Adherence to medication is often very difficult for young people. It is very important that they are supported in this, as stopping medication significantly increases the risk of relapse, usually within the first six months.

Cognitive–Behavioural Therapy (CBT)

CBT has been shown to be helpful for people with Schizophrenia. The person is helped to first identify unhelpful thoughts and behaviours commonly through use of a 'thought record' and 'behaviour diary'. The individual is supported to increase the range of 'healthy' behaviours engaged in, such as exercising, meeting friends or listening to music. The individual is helped to develop a repertoire of alternative more constructive reactions to delusional thoughts and hallucinatory experiences. This can help the individual to develop more control over reactions to psychotic symptoms which in turn lessen the distress associated with these experiences.

Family Work

It is very important that the families of young people with Schizophrenia receive support. A recent study in Dublin has found that involvement in a Family Education Programme can decrease the risk of relapse four-fold. The aim of working with families is to help them to develop a better understanding of their child's illness and how it is treated. For example, parents may find it very useful to focus on early signs of relapse specific to their child, so that they can seek help at the earliest sign of relapse.

Parents often struggle with feelings of guilt after their children are diagnosed, perhaps blaming themselves for their child's illness. It is very important that parents are given the opportunity to address these worries and receive reassurance that families do not cause Schizophrenia.

The focus of family work is usually on practical issues that arise for a family after diagnosis. The aim is to try to provide support for the family and decrease stress.

Myths about Schizophrenia

Schizophrenia is a split personality
The word Schizophrenia is often wrongly used to describe people who are very changeable or to describe something which is difficult to understand 'the committee reached the schizophrenic decision....'

People with schizophrenia are very dangerous
It is rare that young people with schizophrenia are dangerous to others. The risk of violence is increased with using alcohol or street drugs as with the general population. People with schizophrenia are far more vulnerable to being harmed by others than being violent to others.

Schizophrenia never gets better
Twenty per cent of people with Schizophrenia get completely better.

Resources

Shine: 38 Blessington Street Dublin 7; Information Helpline: 1890 621 631;
  Telephone : 01-8601620 e-mail: info@sirl.ie
  Website: www.shineonline.ie; www.recover.ie

Rethink, Head Office, 30 Tabernacle Street, London, EC2A 4DD.
  Tel: 0044 20 7330 9100. UK voluntary organisation that helps people with any
  severe mental illness, their families and carers.
  www.rethink.orgYoung People's site: www.rethink.org/at-ease

Mind, Granta House, 15-19 Broadway, London E15 4BQ;
  Tel: 0044 20 8519 2122
  Fax: 020 8522 1725
  Email: info@mind.org.uk
  Website: www.mind.org.uk
  Publishes a wide range of literature on all aspects of mental health.

12 Stress in Children

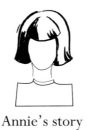

Annie's story

Annie is in first year at school, having joined the class late in the academic year as she had moved from another area. The reason for her move was the recent separation of her parents. School exams are commencing in two weeks. Annie's academic performance and social skills do not appear to fit with those described by her previous teacher. She is struggling to make friends in contrast to the 'bubbly, popular child' described in school reports from her previous school. Annie frequently appears tense and anxious...

What is Stress?

Stress occurs when a person perceives that the challenge they face exceeds their capacity to cope. The demands are known as 'stressors' and the result is the 'stress response'. Stressors can be acute (sudden) or chronic (long lasting).

Is stress good or bad?

Hans Selye was one of the original researchers on stress. Selye (1956) described stress as 'not necessarily something bad - it all depends on how you take it. The stress of exhilarating, creative successful work is beneficial, while that of failure, humiliation or infection is detrimental'.

Today we view stress as normal, and something almost everyone experiences. The majority of children will have experienced stress long before they reach adulthood. Children may have had to cope with family conflict, separation, bullying, exam pressure, domestic violence and violence in their wider communities.

Children who learn to cope with stressful situations can build resilience and in some situations coping with stressors such as an important exam, can give a sense of achievement. In addition, many stressors can lead to a young person developing coping strategies which help them to deal with adversity later in life. However depending on the individual child, chronic stress may have a significant negative impact on well-being. Chronic stress can lead to low self-esteem, depression, suicidal thinking and anxiety disorders. Furthermore it can lead to poor academic performance thereby preventing a child from reaching full potential. Physical health can also be compromised by chronic stress.

Why do young people respond to stress differently?

The level of stress experienced by each child depends on the individual's perception of the stressor. This perception will in turn be influenced by a range of factors; some intrinsic to the child such as personality, maturity and coping style and others reflecting extrinsic factors such as parental support or support in the community.

The personal factors which may help to protect against stress include self-esteem, temperament (the child's type of personality) and good physical health. The young person's belief in a 'locus of control' is a very important influence on the impact of stress. 'Locus of control' may be internal or external. Someone with an internal locus of control believes that they have the capacity to influence what happens to them and respond better to stress. Those with an external locus of control believe that they cannot change or shape events, see these events as inevitable and tend to respond less favourably to stressful situations.

The child's developmental age will impact on the perception of stressful. A younger child may be less prone to stress in certain circumstances due to a lack of understanding (a parent losing a job), while an older child might be more liable to worry about possible consequences in this scenario. In other situations being older might buffer the effects of the stressor as the child has more life-experience to help them manage the situation. Children with below average IQ are also more likely to have difficulties coping with stress. The child's ability to cope will also be a function of the duration and intensity of the stressor.

The impact of a stressor on a young person is highly dependent on the degree of support available to them from family, friends and teachers. Studies with families who have experienced the trauma of war and natural disasters such as earthquakes have shown that the response of parents to the stress is extremely important in influencing how their child will cope. Parents need to be very mindful of how their own stress impacts on their children. For example, if high stress levels are contributing to marital conflict, the child can be very confused and anxious and more liable to begin to feel under stress.

What is the biological response to stress?

The early research on stress established that the body responds to stressors with a 'fight or flight response'. This response occurs in all organisms and its function can be seen from an evolutionary viewpoint as promoting the survival of the species. When an organism perceives a threat, it releases hormones such as noradrenaline and cortisol. These hormones act throughout the body. In humans, as in other animals, the blood supply is diverted from skin and stomach to the heart and brain. The work of the heart is increased and the increased heart rate and blood pressure allow the heart to pump more blood to muscles. This in turn allows the person to run faster or fight harder. In addition, these hormones ensure that the person's focus is maintained on the threat. The net effect of this physiological response is to increase the likelihood that the person will survive the threat. These responses also occur as a reaction to minor stresses but to a much less marked degree. Consequently they are not usually noticed by the individual in the context of everything else that may be happening in the stressful situation.

While the body's physiological response may be useful in situations where the ultimate aim is survival, it is much less useful in dealing with other stressors. The release of this cascade of hormones causes people to feel more irritable, jumpy and anxious. Performance on tasks that require concentration may be compromised by a racing heart and shaking hands. The increased focus on the stressor may also be unhelpful in drawing the person's attention away from other sources of information that might in fact help them to cope better with the 'stressor'. Furthermore, when a hormone such as cortisol is released chronically in response to ongoing stress, it may lead to depression and helplessness. In many cases therefore, the negative impact of the 'fight or flight' response may outweigh the positive.

What are the benefits of stress?

A certain amount of anxiety can be helpful. For example, prior to an exam anxiety can act as a catalyst to students to make extra efforts with their study. However, anxiety only improves performance up to a certain critical point. When anxiety levels start to escalate beyond a certain threshold there is a fall off in performance ability. This is known as the Yerkes-Dodson Law.

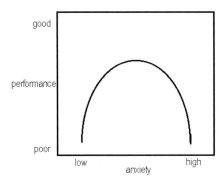

Fig. 12.1   Performance - Anxiety

What are the negative effects of stress?

Stress can have a negative impact on a young person's physical well-being, ability to regulate emotions, relationships with others and mental functioning. Stress can also act as a precipitant to psychiatric illness.

Stress can have a wide-range of physical effects. Children may experience stomach aches and generalised aches and pains as a result of their stress-levels. Stress can also exacerbate medical conditions such as asthma, colitis and migraine.

The young person who is stressed may become much more prone to anger and aggressive outbursts, may appear persistently irritable and some may become depressed. The impact of stress on a young person's emotional regulation can lead to strained relationships with parents and friends, which may in effect isolate them further from sources of support.

Stress can also lead to the young person having difficulty with concentration and consequently having difficulty remembering things. School-work can become very demanding in this context. The child who is experiencing stress, from whatever source, may find that it requires immense additional effort to perform academically. Finally, psychiatric disorders such as an Acute Stress Reaction and Post-Traumatic Stress Disorder may occur as a result of stress.

What signs should the teacher look out for?

Psychological

➤ Difficulty concentrating;
➤ Distractibility;
➤ Inability to finish tasks;
➤ Feeling unable to cope;
➤ Crying very readily;
➤ Appearing constantly tired and lacking energy;
➤ Persistent Irritability;
➤ Anger outbursts and 'flying off the handle';
➤ Loss of sense of humour.

Physical
➤ Change in appetite - decreased or craving for food;
➤ Indigestion, heartburn, nausea, vomiting;

> Change in sleep pattern;
> Muscular twitching, appearing agitated and restless;
> Headaches;
> Breathlessness;
> Skin rashes.

What are the Risk Factors for coping poorly with stress?

> Individual history of psychiatric illness;
> Chronic physical illness;
> Experience of abuse;
> Family dysfunction;
> Family history of depression, deliberate self-harm, alcohol abuse.

How do young people cope with stress?

The different approaches of coping with stress can be broken into two broad categories: problem focused coping and emotion focused coping. The 'problem focused coping style' is an active approach where the young person is on the offensive to tackle the situation: evaluating the available information, making a decision and confronting the problem. The individual attempts to change the stressful situation into a less stressful alternative. The 'emotion focused' style of coping is reactive rather than active. The young person is 'on the defensive' against the stress, attempting to minimise the impact of the stress as opposed to changing the stressor.

What can teachers do to help?

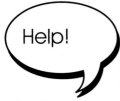

It is important to attempt to make the school environment as minimally stressful as possible, particularly for those children whose home-life is stressful. A stress-free environment is based on social support, problem-solving and learning to anticipate stress.

Social support can be built up in a number of ways, involving teachers, family and friends. It is important to notice the child who is under pressure, to acknowledge feelings and to praise effort.

Problem-solving is a very useful skill to help young people cope with stress and can be acquired. One useful approach is to practice problem-solving in the class, using the following four questions as the basis:

> ➢ What am I supposed to do?
> ➢ What is my plan, or the alternatives?
> ➢ How is my plan working and why is it not?
> ➢ How did I do?

Myths about Stress

Stress is the same for all children.
Stress is different for every young person. What is stressful to one person may be enjoyable to another. Everyone's response to stress is different.

Stress is always bad for you.
"Stress can be the spice of life or the kiss of death". Stress is a normal part of life. What is important is that children are supported to manage stress so that it does not overwhelm them.

Stress is everywhere so you can't do anything about it.
Many situations may be potentially stressful. Effective stress management helps the young person to look at their situation, explore their goals, set priorities and plan how to achieve them. When stress is not managed in this way, the young person can feel surrounded by 'stressors' and 'prioritising' can seem a very difficult task.

No symptoms, no stress.
Frequently the signs of stress may go unnoticed to the person themselves and those around them. In addition the symptoms may be vague or may be mistaken for another problem.

Only major symptoms of stress require attention.
The early signs of stress are an indication that the young person is finding it difficult to cope and is in need of some support and guidance as to how best to cope with a particular situation.

Resources

The YoungMinds Parents' Information Service provides information and advice on child mental health issues. 102-108 Clerkenwell Road, London EC1M 5SA. Parents' Information Service 0800 018 2138; www.youngminds.org.uk

www.teenagehelathfreak.org.Teenage Health Websites Limited is a web-based site which provides accurate and reliable health information for teenagers.

www.rethink.org/ Rethink, the leading national mental health membership charity, works to help everyone affected by severe mental illness recover a better quality of life. Postal address: Rethink, Head Office, 15th Floor, 89 Albert Embankment, London, SE1 7TP. Tel: 0845 456 0455 email: info@rethink.org

www.peersupport.ukobservatory.com. A web-based magazine, that aims to disseminate the most recent research and practice in the field of peer support.
Marilyn Warner,
European Institute of Health and Medical Sciences,
Duke of Kent Building,
University of Surrey,
Guildford,
Surrey,
GU2 7TE
Tel: 01483 684552
E-mail: marilyn@ukobservatory.com

www.bbc.co.uk/health/mental. This BBC health website is provided for general information only.

www.channel4.com/health/stress

www.themindgym.com The Mind Gym Ltd., 2 Kensington Square, London, W8 5EP UK. Tel: work +44 (0)20 7376 0626

13 Substance Abuse

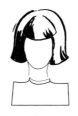

Katie's story

Katie is a fourteen-year-old third year student who has been struggling with schoolwork since first year. Her work has deteriorated significantly recently. Her concentration has noticeably disimproved and she is very irritable with peers and teachers whom she seems to have alienated. On a number of occasions teachers have suspected she has been 'stoned' in class. Up to three months ago, there had not been any significant concerns regarding her behaviour. However, she was recently caught as a passenger in a stolen car and has been allocated a Juvenile Liaison Officer. Attempts by the school to bring their suspicions to the attention of Katie's parents have resulted in her parents threatening to 'throw Katie out of the house'...

What is substance abuse?

Many teenagers experiment with drugs and alcohol. For the vast majority, it does not become a problem. However, a small but significant minority of young people move from experimentation to the point where their use of drugs or alcohol has a significant negative impact on their lives.

How is Substance Abuse Diagnosed?

There are three-broad categories of substance related disorders:
> Substance Abuse
> Substance Dependence
> Substance Induced Disorder

Substance Abuse:

This is a maladaptive pattern of substance use that results in repeated and significant negative consequences for the young person. This may include problems in any domain of the young person's life. Failure to work appropriately at school may compromise relationships with family and friends.

DSM Criteria for Substance Abuse

A. A maladaptive pattern of substance use leading to clinically significant impairment or distress, as manifested by one (or more) of the following, occurring within a 12-month period:

- recurrent substance use resulting in a failure to fulfill major role obligations at work, school, or home (e.g., repeated absences or poor work performance related to substance use; substance-related absences, suspensions, or expulsions from school; neglect of children or household)
- recurrent substance use in situations in which it is physically hazardous (e.g., driving an automobile or operating a machine when impaired by substance use)
- recurrent substance-related legal problems (e.g., arrests for substance-related disorderly conduct)
- continued substance use despite having persistent or recurrent social or interpersonal problems caused or exacerbated by the effects of the substance (e.g., arguments with spouse about consequences of intoxication, physical fights)

B. The symptoms have never met the criteria for Substance Dependence for this class of substance.

Reprinted with permission from The Diagnostic and Statistical Manual of Mental Disorders, Text Revision, Fourth Edition, (Copyright 2000). American Psychiatric Association.

152

Substance Dependence

This is a pattern of substance use that has escalated to the point that the young person is displaying both physical and psychological signs of dependence. These include 'tolerance': the need for increasing amounts of the substance to achieve the desired effect; 'withdrawal symptoms': unpleasant physical sensations which can be relieved if the person consumes the substance and a stereotyped pattern of substance use in which the substance-seeking and substance use take precedence in the young person's life.

DSM Criteria for Substance Dependence

A maladaptive pattern of substance use, leading to clinically significant impairment or distress, as manifested by three (or more) of the following, occurring at any time in the same 12-month period:

- (1) tolerance, as defined by either of the following:
  (a) a need for markedly increased amounts of the substance to achieve intoxication or desired effect
  (b) markedly diminished effect with continued use of the same amount of the substance
- (2) Withdrawal, as manifested by either of the following:
  (a) the characteristic withdrawal syndrome for the substance (refer to Criteria A and B of the criteria sets for Withdrawal from the specific substances)
  (b) the same (or a closely related) substance is taken to relieve or avoid withdrawal symptoms
- (3) the substance is often taken in larger amounts or over a longer period than was intended
- (4) there is a persistent desire or unsuccessful efforts to cut down or control substance use
- (5) a great deal of time is spent in activities necessary to obtain the substance (e.g., visiting multiple doctors or driving long distances), use the substance (e.g., chain-smoking), or recover from its effects
- (6) important social, occupational, or recreational activities are given up or reduced because of substance use
- (7) the substance use is continued despite knowledge of having a persistent or recurrent physical or psychological problem that is likely to have been caused or exacerbated by the substance (e.g., current cocaine use despite recognition of cocaine-induced depression, or continued drinking despite recognition that an ulcer was made worse by alcohol consumption)

Reprinted with permission from The Diagnostic and Statistical Manual of Mental Disorders, Text Revision, Fourth Edition, (Copyright 2000). American Psychiatric Association.

Substance Induced Disorder

This diagnosis describes a physical or mental illness that is the direct consequence of the substance use such as Substance Induced Psychosis. To meet criteria for this disorder, the symptoms should remit approximately one month after the substance use has stopped.

What are the basic drug classes?

- Alcohol
- Amphetamines (speed)
- Caffeine
- Marijuana (grass)
  Cocaine
- Hallucinogens (LSD, ecstasy)
- Inhalants (poppers, glue, solvents)
- Nicotine
- Opioids (heroin, morphine)
  Phencylidine (PCP, angel dust)
- Sedatives (Valium)
  Others: including less common substances and over the counter medications

How common is it?

Regrettably, alcohol and drug use among teens is common. The first phase is typically 'recreational use' and most young people will pass through this phase of experimentation without significant harmful consequence. However, in some cases recreational use may lead to bingeing, which can in turn lead to abuse and dependence. Furthermore, links exist between binge drinking and abuse of other substances. Research has shown that under-age binge drinkers are seven times more likely to have used illicit drugs in the past month than teenagers who do not binge drink. In addition, young people are experimenting with drugs and alcohol earlier than in previous decades. For example, the average age of first using marijuana is fourteen years and many children are experimenting with alcohol at age twelve.

The European School Survey Project on Alcohol and other Drugs study (ESPAD, 2009), which was based on students who turned 16 during the calendar year of data collection reported the following:

* 78% of Irish students had been drinking during the past 12 months
* 47% had been drunk over the same time-scale
* 20% of students had used marijuana/cannabis (twice the European average)
* 15% had used inhalants (almost twice the European average)
* 10% had used illicit drugs other than cannabis
* 7% had used alcohol in combination with tablets
* 3% had used tranquillisers without a prescription

It is important to note that this survey relied on the teenagers' own report so it is likely that it may be an under-estimate of their actual habits. These figures demonstrate that binge drinking is common among Irish teenagers. It is important to view these figures in the context of teenagers from other countries. Compared to other European teenagers, Irish teenagers demonstrate a slightly lower rate of alcohol use in the previous year (78% versus 82%). However, the difference between Irish teenagers and the European average is more marked when comparing the rates of drunkenness. 47% of Irish teenagers reported being drunk in the past year as opposed to 39% of their European peers.

The ESPAD study established that Irish teenagers are as likely to use cannabis as their European counterparts (20 versus 19%). The use of inhalants is higher than the European average (15% versus 9%). The use of street drugs other than cannabis is slightly more common in Irish teenagers (10% versus 7%).

What are the Risk Factors ?

Any child who has access to alcohol and illicit substances could go on to develop substance-related problems. The risk is best understood as a 'risk spectrum'. The more risk factors a young person has, the more likely substance use is to become problematic. The risk is particularly high with drugs which have a high potential for tolerance and withdrawal such as cocaine and heroin.

The following are known to increase a young person's risk of substance misuse:

> * A family history of substance misuse
> * Early school failure
> * Learning difficulties
> * Peer group using drugs
> * Behavioural problems as a child.
> * Untreated ADHD.
> * Poor impulse control.
> * Low self-esteem
> * Family stresses

The influence of genetics is strong and substance-misuse problems frequently run in families. The genetic link has been shown by research that has looked at children of an alcoholic parent who have been adopted and reared by parents without alcohol problems. These studies have shown that adopted children still go on to have significantly greater rates of alcohol problems than children with no family history of alcohol misuse. Family history represents a risk factor which cannot be changed. Fortunately, however, other risk factors are modifiable, for example, poor self esteem, peer group, ADHD and learning difficulties. The ease of access to illicit substances is another modifiable factor which can be influenced by price and cultural attitudes. Furthermore, these risk factors all interact with each other to produce a 'cumulative risk'. Therefore modifying one risk factor can have a significant impact on the overall risk.

What signs should teachers look out for?

Keep in mind that these signs are non-specific and may be signs of other problems as well.
➢ The single strongest indicator is a young person whose best friend uses drugs;
➢ Noticeable deterioration in concentration;
➢ A decline in school performance. The change in academic performance may not be marked;
➢ Increasing discipline problems;

➤ Frequent tardiness and absences;

➤ Appearing drunk or hung-over in class;

➤ Irritability and hypersensitivity. Likely to avoid or deflect questions if confronted;

➤ Trouble with the law;

➤ Shoplifting, stealing from classmates;

➤ If the young person suddenly has new expensive possessions out of keeping with their financial circumstances, it may be an indication of drug-dealing;

➤ Physical signs such as fatigue, repeated health complaints, red and glazed eyes and a persistent cough.

What can the teacher do to help?

It is helpful to have very clear school policies on substance abuse. All students should be aware of school policy and it should be uniformly applied. Schools should adopt a zero-tolerance policy to drug and alcohol use. This does not mean that children should be expelled. However, turning 'a blind eye' to substance misuse is inadvisable. Schools are best advised to develop mandatory guidelines, which are followed in all cases. Similarly, it is imperative to have a school policy for students who are suspected of dealing drugs to other students. If drug or significant alcohol use is identified, parents should be contacted and advised to discuss this with their GP and a referral to local CAMHS or addiction services should be considered.

How could teachers discuss Substance Misuse with teenagers?

It can be helpful to have an open discussion exploring with students their perspectives on why young people might take drugs. This facilitates a realistic discussion which acknowledges that from a user's perspective there are positive consequences of using substances, for example, relaxation or peer acceptance. However, it is important that the discussion emphasizes the fuller picture elaborating the potential negative outcomes of substance-misuse.

Examples of Student responses and possible discussion points:

Peer pressure: 'Everyone else enjoys themselves. I can't be the only one not to join in'

Possible discussion points:

Does it help to always do what everyone else does?

When might this not be helpful?

Are there other ways of 'fitting in?

What are potential downsides of using a 'prop' to fit in?

Are you then more or less likely to use something else you didn't think you would?

Short-term high: 'I feel so relaxed after I've smoked a joint'

Possible discussion points:

How does it feel to be relaxed?

What other ways can people relax?

Why is it helpful to have ways of coping with stress?

Is it likely that the same amount of substance will keep making you relaxed? What happens then?

What do you do?

Confidence. 'I can't deal with my family without a drink.

Discussion points:

What does 'confidence' feel like? How does it help? Are there other ways to feel confident? How might you make a plan to help you cope with what's annoying you about your family? Is drinking a good long-term solution to this problem? Why what's likely to happen? Is this pattern likely to be repeated in other situations? What's a better solution?

Self-medication: 'It helps me to feel happy and to forgot all the things that bother me for a while'.

Discussion points:

Do most people feel sad sometimes? Do a lot of people have worries? What can you do if you feel like that? Is trying to make something disappear the best way to deal with it? Why? What happens if you feel sad again? Is it a good way of learning to cope? Why? What else can you do? How do you plan that?

It can also be useful to explore with students the risks and dangers of drug use:

- ➢ Dangers of mixing drugs and alcohol, e.g. dehydration associated with alcohol and ecstasy;
- ➢ Dangers of not knowing mix of drugs, e.g. drug may be more potent than you realise;
- ➢ Increased likelihood of arguments, fights and accidents;
- ➢ Increased likelihood of mental health difficulties including suicidal thoughts and behaviours;
- ➢ Liver damage;
- ➢ Difficulty concentrating and irritability;
- ➢ Serious infections such as Hepatitis and HIV from needle sharing.

The questions listed below may help the young person to consider the impact of substance abuse. If the student answers 'yes' to these questions it is likely that a problem exists.

- ➢ Do you think about drugs or alcohol every day?
- ➢ Is it difficult to say 'no' when someone offers you drugs/alcohol?
- ➢ Do you use drugs/alcohol when you're alone?
- ➢ Does using/drugs or alcohol seem to take up a lot of your free time?

It is helpful if young people recognise their difficulties. It can be instructive to explore concepts such as 'loss of control' and 'tolerance' to encourage the young person to consider the effect of drug use. For example, if the young person decides not to use drugs, can the substance 'control' the outcome leading to relapse? Is more and more of the substance required to achieve the same effect?

Treatment

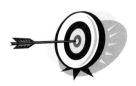

All agencies that work with young people who misuse substances are not the same, nor are the treatments they offer. The type of treatment offered is typically decided on the basis of the severity of the problem and the needs of the individual child. For this reason, the initial assessment is critical to establish the nature and severity of the problem.

The treatment offered is most commonly on an outpatient basis. The therapeutic approach is commonly based on a 'motivational interviewing' style which seeks to harness the young person's own motivation to promote change. The young person may be at any stage of the 'Stages of Change' model. This will depend on multiple factors including, awareness of the problem and its effects in addition to the strength of desire to bring about change. Therapy focuses on trying to move the young person through the 'Stages of Change', seeking an acknowledgment of difficulties and a recognition of the need to change, how change can be achieved and finally how to maintain healthier behaviour.

Stages of Change Model:
   Precontemplation: the person has no awareness that substance use is problematic.
   Contemplation: The person is beginning to consider that substance use may have negative consequences.
   Determination/Preparation: The person is actively considering how to deal with the problem.
   Action: The person changes behaviour in some way to deal with substance misuse.
   Maintenance: The person attempts to maintain healthier behaviour
   Relapse: The person begins to engage in previous harmful patterns of use.

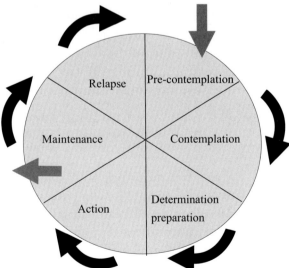

Fig. 13.1   Stages of Change Model

Other forms of therapy that may be useful in helping young people with substance misuse problems include CBT and Family Therapy. Families frequently struggle to know how to cope with their child's behaviour. Providing support to parents is a crucial aspect of treatment.

Generally, medication is only required infrequently with teenagers in severe cases such as heroin addiction. If a young person has developed a chemical dependence, inpatient admission for detoxification may be required. Methadone may be given as a substitute for heroin. Medication may also be necessary to deal with short-term withdrawal effects. If the young person is assessed to have any underlying or additional mental health difficulties, specific medication may also be required. Medication may also be necessary to treat substance induced disorders such as psychoses following cannabis or amphetamine use.

Resources

American Council for Drug Education
  www.acde.org

Alliance for Children and Families
  www.alliance1.org

Drug Enforcement Administration (DEA)
  www.dea.gov

Join Together Online (JTO)
  www.jointogether.org

National Institute on Alcohol Abuse and Alcoholism (NIAAA)
  www.niaaa.nih.gov

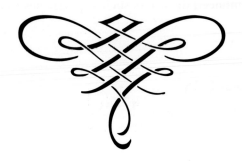

14 Obsessive Compulsive Disorder

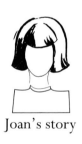

Joan's story

Joan was a 9 year old girl in third class who became quiet and withdrawn in school and seemed to be very slow at completing all her academic tasks. She confided in her teacher that when writing she had to write every seventh word out seven times before she could write the next word. If she stopped before her homework was completed she had to start at the beginning again. This lasted for hours. If she ever touched someone as she passed them she needed to touch them back twice immediately or she would become very distressed. She could not explain why she had to do this, knew it was "silly", but did not "feel right" until she did it...

What is Obsessive Compulsive Disorder (OCD)?

OCD is a disorder characterised by recurrent intrusive thoughts, images and impulses or compulsive behaviours that cause marked distress and/or interference in a person's life.

The DSM –IV Diagnosis of Obsessive compulsive Disorder is based on the following characteristic symptoms

Either obsessions or compulsions:

Obsessions are defined by:
- recurrent and persistent thoughts, impulses, or images that are experienced, at some time during the disturbance, as intrusive and inappropriate and that cause marked anxiety or distress
- the thoughts, impulses, or images are not simply excessive worries about real-life problems
- the person attempts to ignore or suppress such thoughts, impulses, or images, or to neutralize them with some other thought or action
- the person recognizes that the obsessional thoughts, impulses or images are a product of his or her own mind (not imposed from without as in thought insertion).

Compulsions as defined by:
- repetitive behaviours (e.g., hand washing, ordering, checking) or mental acts (e.g., praying, counting, repeating words silently) that the person feels driven to perform in response to an obsession, or according to rules that must be applied rigidly. The behaviours or mental acts are aimed at preventing or reducing distress or preventing some dreaded event or situation; however, these behaviours or mental acts either are not connected in a realistic way with what they designed to neutralize or prevent or are clearly excessive.

Reprinted with permission from The Diagnostic and Statistical Manual of Mental Disorders, Text Revision, Fourth Edition, (Copyright 2000). American Psychiatric Association.

How is Obsessive Compulsive Disorder diagnosed?

Many young children (and indeed adults) have some obsessional behaviour such as not standing on cracks, not allowing themselves walk under ladders or always needing to sleep with a certain object. Many of these are superstitions and are carried out or adhered to to avoid some unpleasant event or consequence, such as bad luck after walking under a ladder. These behaviours are developmentally appropriate, generally decrease as the child gets older and do not cause significant upset. Some individuals may continue to be somewhat obsessional as they grow older - putting items away in a predefined order, fastidious cleaning, attention to detail. Such behaviour is benign and may be beneficial.

Obsessional thoughts or behaviours that lead to significant distress and interfere significantly with the individual's emotional, academic or family life are characteristic of OCD. Obsessions can be in the form of involuntary thoughts, urges or impulses. The main features of obsessions are that they are frequent, automatic and very anxiety provoking. Obsessions commonly include a fear of dirt, germs, fear of acting violently or an unreasonable fear of harming others.

Compulsions are rituals that a child feels compelled to carry out. It is common for people to carry out a compulsion in order to reduce anxiety experienced from obsessive thoughts. Compulsions can be observable actions such as excessive hand washing or mental rituals such as repeating certain words, counting or praying.

What signs should teachers look out for?

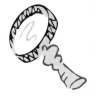

> Children may repeatedly wash their hands to prevent 'something bad happening';
> Some children may avoid certain situations or seek reassurance repeatedly;
> The child may become very anxious if the compulsion is not carried out. The following are common compulsions: repeating actions including: checking, touching, counting, ordering and arranging;
> A child handing in homework late which may have been rubbed out or corrected excessively;
> A need to have things 'just right', a need for symmetry when washing, walking, or touching.

What are the effects of OCD?

OCD can cause severe disruptions to academic performance, peer relationships and family functioning. Family members often become involved in maintaining the rituals of the OCD. For example, a child may repeatedly ask parents for reassurance regarding 'cleanliness'. This can culminate in parents becoming participants in elaborate rituals such as washing the child in a certain way for hours at a time, according to certain 'rules'. The OCD can become so dominant in a child's life that going out with friends is avoided due to time spent on rituals. Children with compulsions about cleaning may end up with sores and excoriations due to repeated washing. Parents may feel increasingly helpless as to how to prevent the behaviour from escalating or may react to demands to participate in rituals in different ways, which can lead to increased tension in the family.

Can anyone develop OCD?

Approximately 1 in 200 children and adolescents develop OCD. However, many children are ashamed and keep their symptoms of OCD a secret so the rates may be higher. Research has demonstrated that OCD is more common in boys with a ratio of approximately 2:1 (male to female).

Is OCD a 'new phenomenon'?

OCD has been described since the 17th century, when obsessions and compulsions were often described as being associated with religious melancholy. The Oxford Don, Robert Burton reported a case in his compendium, "The Anatomy of Melancholy" of a man who was afraid that he would unintentionally speak 'indecent thoughts' out loud. In the 19th century modern concepts of OCD evolved.

What causes OCD?

 In some cases OCD may be linked with an underlying biochemical imbalance. It is thought that there may be insufficient levels of the chemical serotonin in the brain. However, this does not fully explain the symptoms.

OCD can occur as a result of streptococcal infections. This is called "Paediatric Autoimmune Neuropsychiatric Disorders Associated with

Streptococcal infections" or PANDAS. OCD may also occur with various neurological conditions including brain tumours, carbon monoxide poisoning, post-viral encephalitis, or rarely, an allergic reaction to a wasp sting.

Genetic Factors

The tendency to develop this disorder involves complex genetic and environmental factors. At least 50% of children with Pteriidae's Syndrome (a disorder characterised by both motor and vocal tics) develop obsessive compulsive symptoms by adulthood. 60% of children with OCD have a history of Tics (see Chapter 11). First degree relatives show an increased rate of Tic and OCD disorders based on twin and family studies. This implies that there is a definite genetic component in some cases of OCD and a link between OCD and Tic Disorders.

Familial Factors

Research suggests that in some cases children with OCD come from families where parents are somewhat over-involved in managing their children. The home environment may be very tightly controlled. It is hypothesised that some children display similar behaviours to parents who may have obsessive traits themselves. Therefore, in these cases the link may be genetic or the child's OCD may have developed in the context of modelling from parents. Parents do not cause OCD in their children as the development of the illness is multifactorial.

Cultural Factors

OCD occurs in all cultures but is reported to be more common in Caucasian children. The reasons for this are unknown.

What can the teacher do to help?

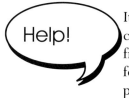

It is important to remember that most children with OCD can become extremely anxious and distressed if prevented from engaging in compulsive behaviour. The child may feel compelled to engage in specific rituals or routines to prevent distress and these compulsions may be disruptive to the class.

It is often helpful to encourage relaxation exercises for the class. It is very useful to try to identify triggers in classroom or school yard that may make a child with OCD more anxious. This can be done by keeping a note of times when the child appears distressed, looking for trends and considering what may have precipitated the child's anxiety at these particular times. For example, a child may become more upset in the lead up to break-time on a repeated basis. If this pattern is noted, it may be worth exploring with the child whether there is anything about break-time that is upsetting. It can be very useful to then help the child to problem-solve ways in which break-time can become more manageable.

OCD also takes up a lot of a child's energy and time and consequently academic performance may not be at the expected level. If a child is obsessionally slow, encouragement will be required to leave schoolwork undone and to change tasks even if left unfinished. This will help the child learn to switch tasks which can be extremely difficult for someone with OCD.

If a child is spending hours on homework ('having' to have it perfect), written work should be reduced where possible. For primary school children, it is particularly important to work closely with parents to ensure a limit is put on homework time. Many children with obsessions and compulsions related to schoolwork may become extremely distressed which may in turn escalate family tensions. It is important to encourage the child to hand in a series of draft versions of homework thus allowing the child to cope with 'imperfections'.

It is essential to look out for signs of the child becoming distressed and to plan time-outs if necessary. If overwhelmed or unable to complete class-work, the child may need to have an individual daily programme . The most helpful way to do this is often to meet with the child and parents to identify the main areas of difficulty and agree on the important areas that need to be targeted.

If the child feels unable to stop a compulsion it may be helpful to agree to allow the ritual at prescribed times such as lunchtime.

When is professional help needed?

If the child's obsessive thoughts or compulsive behaviours are impairing social, academic or family functioning, professional help may be required.

Parents should be contacted and advised to bring the child to their GP initially who will then refer to CAMHS if appropriate.

Treatment

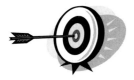

Education and support are very important for the child, parents and teachers. The child should have a full medical examination to rule out any medical cause for OCD. Following this a child should be referred to the local CAMHS team or psychology service for treatment. It is important to watch out for Depression or Tic Disorders as often young people have more than one disorder. Usually the treatment is carried out in an outpatient department. However, if a child is extremely distressed by symptoms or very impaired in everyday life, more intensive input from a Child and Adolescent Day Hospital or an inpatient unit may be necessary.

Cognitive Behavioural Therapy

Cognitive Behavioural Therapy is the treatment of choice for children with OCD as research studies have established its effectiveness. Therapy typically begins with a detailed assessment of the thoughts and behaviours which are problematic. This may be done by the child and family keeping a diary of obsessions and compulsions. Each obsession and compulsion is then placed into a 'hierarchy'. The place of each symptom on the hierarchy is based on the distress the child experiences in response to the specific obsession or compulsion.

Frequently the next step in therapy is to teach the child how to identify anxious feelings and how to use relaxation techniques and deep breathing. This will prepare the child for the next step and allow the child to participate in various "behaviour experiments" which are crucial to the successful management of OCD. For example, if a child has a fear of germs, 'germs' must be faced in multiple guises. This is organised in a stepwise fashion. The child may first have to think about germs and then draw germs and finally build up to touching a feared 'dirty' object. At each step, the child is supported to overcome anxiety and helped not to engage in compulsive behaviour (despite the anxiety this provokes). Learning how to confront the anxiety caused by engaging in compulsive behaviours is key to treating symptoms of OCD. The child is helped to develop a 'toolkit' which consists of alternative positive coping strategies which can be utilised when experiencing an obsession or compulsion.

Medication

A child who is not responding to CBT may need medication. A number of studies have shown that for moderate or severe OCD, the best treatment is a combined approach using both medication and CBT. The medications that are useful in treating OCD act in the brain to increase a chemical called serotonin. Most commonly either Fluoxetine (Prozac) or Sertraline (Lustral) is used; these are also used to treat Depression. Many children do not show an improvement in their obsessive compulsive symptoms until they are on the medication for six weeks.

Family Work

Parents are advised to help children not to become involved in elaborate time consuming rituals. They can help children use distraction and relaxation techniques. Some children become very distressed if they are interrupted carrying out their ritual. Families need to be careful that they do not become extensively involved either in the child's compulsive rituals or in reassuring the child's obsessional worries as parents may inadvertently perpetuate the child's behaviour. It is important to try and maintain a calm and supportive environment.

Myths

OCD does not exist. It is just people being fussy and they are just looking for attention.
It is extremely common to have a few obsessional thoughts or minor compulsions. However the obsessive thoughts and compulsive actions of OCD severely disrupt people's lives.

People with OCD are just quirky and could stop this behaviour if they want to.
OCD is not a matter of willpower and people do not just choose to behave in a certain way. Thoughts are overwhelming, compelling the individual to act in particular ways.

Stress causes OCD and if people could relax they would be fine.
Stress may exacerbate OCD but is not the cause of the disorder .

Resources

Useful Websites

Obsessive-Compulsive Anonymous. P.O. Box 215, New Hyde Park, NY 11040.
(516)741-4901. west24th@aol.com
http://members.aol.com/west24th/index.html
info@ocdireland.org

Books

The Sky is Falling: Understanding and Coping with Phobias, Panic and Obsessive-Compulsive Disorders. Dumont, Raeann. New York: W. W. Norton & Co., 1996.

'*Kids Like Me*' - Children's stories about Obsessive Compulsive Disorder, Constance Foster. 1997

Obsessive-Compulsive Foundation. P.O. Box 70, Milford, CT 06460. (203) 874-3843. JPHS28A@Prodigy.com
http://pages.prodigy.com/alwillen/ocf.html

Swedo, S. E., and H. L. Leonard. *It's Not All In Your Head.* New York: HarperCollins, 1996.

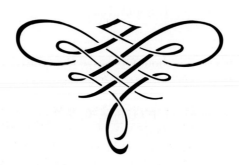

15 Medication: Commonly Used Medication in Young People

Methylphenidate

Methylphenidate, commonly known as Ritalin, is prescribed to treat ADHD. Methylphenidate acts as a Central Nervous System stimulant by increasing levels of the brain chemical dopamine. The effect of this is to improve attention and reduce hyperactivity.

Methylphenidate has been shown conclusively in a very large well-designed study in the USA to result in the best outcomes for children with ADHD in the short-term. The difference between the improvements with medication versus other forms of treatment is, however, less marked over time.

Methylphenidate comes in a number of different forms including Ritalin, Ritalin LA, Equasym and Concerta XL. The main difference between these drugs is their duration of action within the body. Ritalin starts to work after approximately twenty minutes and its effect lasts about 3-4 hours, therefore a child may take it twice or three times a day. Ritalin LA lasts eight to ten hours and Concerta lasts about eight to twelve hours.

Children will be prescribed different types and doses of medication and at different frequencies depending on their symptom profile. The longer acting medications allow simpler dosing regimes (taken once a day) and may improve adherence. Some children are embarrassed by having to take medication at school and the longer acting medications can be helpful in this regard.

The commonest side-effects with Methylphenidate are nervousness and insomnia. Abdominal pain, nausea and vomiting also occur commonly. The young person is monitored regularly in the clinic to check if these side-effects occur. Methylphenidate may have an impact on growth and weight. Therefore, height and weight are regularly measured.

Teachers and parents may be asked to fill out questionnaires a number of times to help the clinician track progress. This is a very useful way of gaining an objective picture of the child's response to medication in different settings.

The length of time that a child remains on medication will vary. The child may be given some time off medication to check if symptoms of ADHD are still evident. It is usually best to time a trial off medication to coincide with an uneventful period in the school year that is not close to exams, holidays or festive occasions.

Atomoxetine HCL

Atomoxetine is a recently licensed drug in Ireland for ADHD. It decreases hyperactivity and improves concentration by increasing the level of the neurotransmitter, noradrenaline, in the brain. Very common side-effects include decreased appetite, abdominal pain and vomiting. Other side-effects that occur commonly include cold/flu symptoms, fatigue, sleep disturbance, mood swings and dizziness. Height and weight are monitored regularly.

The effectiveness of Atomoxetine is measured in the same way as Methylphenidate.

Fluoxetine

The trade-name of Fluoxetine is Prozac; it can be used to treat depression, Obsessive Compulsive Disorder, Anxiety and Bulimia. Fluoxetine is one of a group of medications known as Selective-Serotonin Reuptake Inhibitors (SSRI). As with all SSRIs it works by increasing the levels of serotonin, a naturally occurring substance in the brain. SSRI medications are better tolerated than older antidepressants as they have fewer side-effects. Furthermore, they cause fewer problems if taken as an overdose, which is a risk in young people known to be depressed.

Fluoxetine is usually reserved for use in children with more severe forms of depression, OCD or Anxiety. The use of psychological therapies alone may be sufficient in milder forms of these illnesses. Side-effects of Fluoxetine include nausea and diarrhoea, headache, difficulty sleeping, anxiety, restlessness and agitation.

There is evidence that some SSRIs can increase thoughts of suicide in young people who are depressed. This was not found in research studies of Fluoxetine and the benefits of using Fluoxetine have been shown to outweigh any risks associated with it. For this reason, Fluoxetine is the antidepressant of choice when treating moderate to severe depression in young people. Fluoxetine should only be prescribed for young people after a comprehensive assessment by a psychiatrist and should be carefully monitored.

Fluoxetine usually takes a number of weeks to improve symptoms. Approximately 60% of young people with depression will respond to treatment with Fluoxetine alone and 70% when it is used in conjunction with Cognitive Behavioural Therapy. It is very difficult to predict, before initiating treatment, which children will respond to medication.

When treating depression, young people should continue to take their medication for at least six months after their symptoms have resolved. The discontinuation of medication should only take place under the supervision of a psychiatrist.

Sertraline

Sertraline is another SSRI. It can be used to treat OCD. It is usually taken once a day in the morning or evening.

It may take eight to ten weeks to result in noticeable effects on symptoms. Approximately 40% of children respond to Sertraline when it is used alone and this figure increases to 53% when used in conjunction with CBT. If one medication is not effective, another type of drug should be tried.

Side effects include upset stomach, nausea, diarrhoea, vomiting, loss of appetite, weight changes, drowsiness, excessive tiredness, difficulty falling asleep or staying asleep, shaking hands, nervousness or excitement. As with all mental health medications, Sertraline should only be discontinued under the supervision of a psychiatrist.

Risperidone

Risperidone belongs to a type of drug called 'atypical' or second-generation antipsychotics. It is used to treat Schizophrenia and is also used in the short-term treatment of Bipolar Affective Disorder (Manic Depression). It can also be used to regulate severe behavioural disturbance and occasionally it is used for this purpose in children with Autism, Learning Disability or other neuro-psychiatric disorders. It works by regulating the activity of two naturally occurring substances in the brain: dopamine and serotonin.

Risperidone is usually introduced at low-doses in order to minimise side-effects and is increased gradually while monitoring response. Side-effects of Risperidone include transient sedation, headache, insomnia, agitation, anxiety and weight gain.

If the young person with psychosis or Schizophrenia does not respond to an adequate dose of Risperidone after a period of approximately 2 months, the medication will usually be changed to another type of antipsychotic. In the longer term, a balance needs to be achieved between the effectiveness of the medication and the tolerability of side-effects.

Olanzapine

Olanzapine is prescribed to young people with Psychosis, Schizophrenia or Bipolar Affective Disorder. Olanzapine is another 'atypical' or second generation antipsychotic which achieves its effect by regulating serotonin and dopamine levels in the brain.

In keeping with best practice with any psychiatric medication, the young person starts on a low dose of Olanzapine which is gradually increased depending on its effectiveness and tolerability.

Side-effects include tiredness, increased appetite, significant weight gain, abnormal muscle movements, stiffness and dizziness. The extent of the side-effects experienced by the young person is monitored and weighed against the effectiveness of the medication in reducing psychotic symptoms. If there is a favourable, risk-benefit profile, the young person will remain on the medication. If not the medication will be changed.

Antipsychotics do not 'cure' Schizophrenia, they treat it, similarly to how insulin treats rather than cures diabetes. In general young people are advised to remain on medication for one to two years after a first episode of psychosis. Relapse is very common, even after this duration of treatment, with up to 80% relapsing when medication is stopped. In the vast majority of cases, long term treatment with antipsychotic medication will be required to control the illness.

Melatonin

Melatonin is a naturally occurring hormone produced in the body in association with the body's circadian rhythm. The natural rise in melatonin which occurs in the evening usually precedes sleep by approximately ninety minutes. Melatonin is commonly prescribed to treat children with sleep difficulties. Up to 80% of children with developmental difficulties and ten percent of children in general have sleep difficulties.

A number of studies have demonstrated an improvement in the time taken for children to fall asleep when prescribed melatonin. However, it has not been consistently demonstrated that there is any overall improvement in the number of times the child wakes overnight or the total amount of sleep.

The side-effects of melatonin includes headache, depression, restlessness, confusion, nausea and increased heart rate.

Benzodiazepines

Benzodiazepines such as Diazepam (Valium) or Alprazolam (Xanax) are rarely used in children. When prescribed in children, benzodiazepines are usually only used when the child is acutely agitated. The use is short-term and the child is very closely monitored.

Alternative Treatments:

Omega–3 Fatty Acids
Omega-3 Fatty acids are polyunsaturated fats. The polyunsaturated fatty acids alpha-linolenic acid (ALA) and linolenic acid (LA) cannot be made by the body and therefore must be obtained in the diet. Omega-3 fatty acids can be obtained in the diet in fish oils, green leafy vegetables, nuts, vegetable oils such as canola, soy and especially flaxseed. The omega-3 fatty acid ALA is converted in the body to eicosapentaenoic acid (EPA) and docosahexaenoic

acid (DHA). Experts agree that individuals should consume more omega-3 and less omega-6 in their diets.

Omega-3 fatty acids are an increasingly popular over-the-counter remedy for a variety of mental and physical health problems in both children and adults. There is not enough reliable evidence available to conclude that omega-3 fatty acids are an effective treatment for mental health difficulties in children, or that they should replace standard treatments. There is one recent study that has indicated that omega-3 fatty acids may be therapeutically effective in childhood depression, however, larger well-designed studies are necessary to substantiate the results of this study. The potential for therapeutic benefit from omega-3 oils in children with neurodevelopmental disorders such as Autism and ADHD is also being explored.

The information on potential side-effects associated with omega-3 oils is incomplete. However, the information available to date suggests that side-effects are uncommon and when they do occur are frequently minor such as gastrointestinal upset.

St. John's Wort

St. John's Wort (Hypericum Perforatum) is an herb which has gained increasing popularity in recent years as an 'alternative' treatment for depression in adults. Although it has been used for centuries as an herbal treatment, there is little scientific knowledge as to its composition or its possible mechanism of action. There are a number of chemicals in the herb. Hypericin and hyperforin are thought to be its active ingredients. Research to date suggests that St. John's Wort may act by preventing the uptake of serotonin in the brain, similar to the mechanism of action of conventional antidepressants. It has also been proposed that it may work through its effect on the immune system. Further research is required to provide clarity as to its mechanism of action.

There have been no scientific trials to establish whether St. John's Wort is effective in treating mental health difficulties in children. Results in adults have been contradictory, with some European studies suggesting it may be effective in mild to moderate depression, whereas studies in the USA have found it no more effective than a placebo. Trials are ongoing to explore whether St. John's Wort may be effective in a range of mental health problems in adults.

The most common side-effects are dry mouth, dizziness, diarrhoea, nausea, light sensitivity and fatigue. St. John's Wort has been shown to interact with immunosuppressants and cancer chemotherapeutic agents.

Herbal agents such as 'St. John's Wort' which are often described as 'natural' may be dangerous if taken in large quantities. It is important that parents of children taking herbal remedies inform their doctor, just as they should with prescribed medication. It is never advised that parents try to medicate children themselves as doing so has multiple potential adverse outcomes.

Myths about using psychiatric medication with children

It is better to 'just wait' for mental health difficulties to pass without medication.
The decision to put a young person on medication is weighed up very carefully and is dependent on a variety of factors. If left without medication, some difficulties may not resolve, others may get more severe and in some cases significant secondary problems can accrue.

Only suicidal children need medication.
The assessment of the need for medication is informed by multiple variables including severity of symptoms, the impairment caused by symptoms and previous response to medication. The assessment of the child's 'suicidality' is one of a range of reasons that a child may be put on medication.

Medications used for children with psychiatric problems are addictive.
The standard medications used in child psychiatry are not habit forming or addictive.

Medications used for children with psychiatric problems change their personalities.
Medications do not change personalities but are used to treat the symptoms of psychiatric illness with the aim of helping the young person feel like themselves again.

It is always better for a young person with mental health difficulties to receive therapy before medication.
The research evidence supports different treatment approaches with different difficulties. In some specific cases, medication is the best first-line treatment.

Resources

National Institute of Mental Health: www.nimh.nih.gov

National Institute of Clinical Excellence: www.nice.org.uk

New York University Child Study Centre www.aboutourkids.org

US Food and Drug Administration: www.fda.gov/

US Department of Health, National Institute of Alternative Medicine
   http://nccam.nih.gov/health

16 Child Development Theory: the historical context

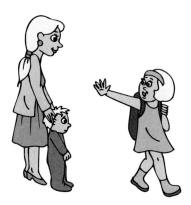

At times the boundary between normal and abnormal behaviour can appear vague. Furthermore what is normal at one age or developmental level may be inappropriate or abnormal at another. Therefore, an understanding of normal child development is essential to an understanding of children's mental health.

Brain Development

Brain development is hugely complex with at least 50% of the entire human genome dedicated to this process. The brain and nervous system develop from embryonic tissue called the ectoderm. The beginning of neural system development occurs at approximately the 16th day of embryonic development, when a mother rarely even knows she is pregnant. The brain grows at a phenomenal rate during intrauterine life with approximately 50,000 cells being added every second for most of this period. Research suggests that sensory awareness begins to develop very early in foetal life. Touch is the first sense to develop at eight weeks, followed by taste at 12 weeks and hearing at 22-24 weeks, while the baby is still in utero. It is thought that the predominant influence on brain development is genetic. However, a myriad of other factors may also influence this process, including the mother's use of alcohol and drugs, in addition to her physical and mental well-being and general state of mind during pregnancy. Recent research also suggests that aspects of the mother's external environment can impact on intrauterine life. For example, newborn infants have been shown to preferentially respond to sounds in the mother's language rather than a foreign language, implying that the developing foetus is being sensitised to external factors during pregnancy.

At birth there is a huge excess of neurons in the infant's brain and these are selectively destroyed in the last month of pregnancy and early postnatal period. The brain continues to grow after birth, predominantly due to the proliferation of glial cells, which are the cells that insulate nerve cells. By the age of two, the brain is approximately 80% of its adult size. The neuronal cells also continue to make many new connections after birth. Connections between neurons are called synapses and it is via synapses that nerve cells communicate. At synapses, neurons release neurotransmitters (brain chemicals) thereby passing on the neural signal to the next cell. Nerve cells can have multiple branches. There may be tens of thousands of synapses at a single neuron looking like a very busy crossroad. This results in trillions of connections throughout the entire nervous system.

Synapse development most likely starts in the mid to late second trimester and continues after birth. This process of synapse formation continues at its peak rate for approximately 6-8 years and then begins to decrease. This process is described as 'pruning', when unnecessary connections are discarded. This is the so-called 'use-it-or lose it' phenomenon which has been demonstrated in animal experiments. For example, experiments have shown that chimpanzees who received no visual stimulation after birth were blind by the age of 6 months. As they had not used their visual tracks, they were discarded and 'lost'. The period of maximal synapse development mirrors the period in which the child is exposed to a vast array of new information early in life. Different parts of the brain seem to develop at different ages. For example, part of the brain which coordinates spatial and language processing show a very significant growth spurt between the ages 6-13 years. The subsequent decrease in growth after this time coincides with the end of the period typically thought of as a critical period for language acquisition.

Recently, it has been recognised that brain development continues into adolescence. Researchers have used brain imaging, where children have had brain scans every two years, to increase our understanding of how the brain continues to develop. Somewhat surprisingly, this research demonstrated that there is a second period of overproduction of neural cells that occurs just prior to adolescence. This process peaks at around 11 years in girls and 12 years in boys. Furthermore, it has been demonstrated that neuronal production in different parts of the adolescent brain peak at different stages consistent with cognitive changes that are occurring at these different times. For example, the peak in growth in neurons that occurs just prior to adolescence is most noticeable in the front part or frontal lobe of the brain. This is the area of the brain that coordinates 'executive function' which includes planning, reasoning and impulse control. Studies have further demonstrated differences between the nerve density and pathways in the frontal lobes of teenagers and those of young adults, again adding weight to the idea that changes in brain structure mirror cognitive shifts that are occurring at these stages.

Diagram of the Brain with Lobes Identified

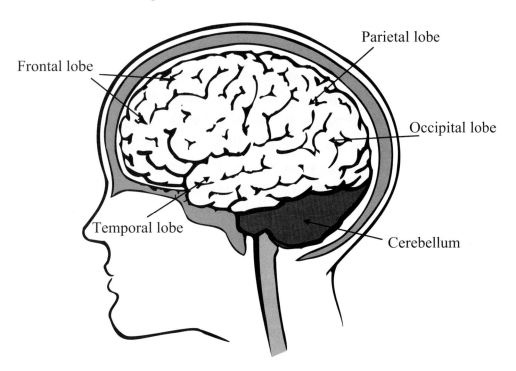

183

In contrast, parts of the brain , which coordinate sensory, spatial and language processing (the parietal and temporal lobes), are almost fully developed by adolescence. Researchers have also demonstrated changes in the brain areas that are activated during certain tasks at different stages of development. For example, when teenagers were shown pictures of faces displaying different emotions while simultaneously imaging their brains, it was noted that there was an increase in brain activity in the amygdala, an area of the brain that processes 'gut reactions'. When the same experiment was carried out with adults, researchers demonstrated increased activity of the frontal lobe implying increased reasoning in the response of adults to emotional stimuli. Thus, as children move from childhood to adolescence to adulthood they use different parts of the brain for the same tasks.

Anatomy of the adult brain

The brain is divided into two non-identical cerebral hemispheres. 90% of people have one dominant hemisphere, usually the left. Cerebral dominance has usually developed by the age of three. At this age the parent may notice that the child prefers to use the right hand to draw for example , the right foot to kick, and the right eye to look through a key hole. The functions of the hemispheres are 'lateralised'. The left hemisphere controls the right side of the body and the right hemisphere controls the left side of the body.

Table 16.1 Functions of Brain Lobes

Specific Functions of Left Hemisphere	Language and Sequencing
Specific Functions of Right Hemisphere	Emotions, Creativity, Music, Imagination, Visuo-spatial ability.
Frontal Lobe	Motor Control Planning of Movement Overall organisation and planning
Temporal Lobe	Memory Auditory Processing
Parietal Lobe	Orientation in Space (i.e. 3 dimensional)
Occipital Lobe	Visual Processing
Cerebellum	Fine Motor Control

Developmental Stages

Developmental Stages have been conceptualised in many different ways since children's development was first studied. A number of different theories are described below.

Freud's Stages of Psychosexual Development

Sigmund Freud (1865-1939), born in Austria, was a neurologist and psychiatrist. He is regarded as the 'father of psychoanalysis'. His legacy is far-reaching and can be seen in literature, literary criticism, film, feminist theory, philosophy and psychology.

Freud credited a colleague, Joseph Breuer, with the discovery of psychoanalysis based on the case of a 21 year-old female, Anna O, which Breuer described to Freud. The young woman was being treated for 'hysterical symptoms' including non-organic paralysis. Breuer noticed that during her hysterical states, Anna mumbled words which he transcribed. Breuer then hypnotised Anna, repeated her words back to her and in the process discovered that these words were related to her father's illness and death. Freud went on to develop this technique and used it with a wide variety of celebrated cases. The goal of psychoanalysis was essentially to bring unconscious or repressed ideas into awareness.

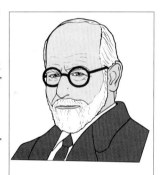

Sigmund Freud
1856-1939

The concept of the 'unconscious' was one of Freud's greatest contributions to modern thinking. Freud described how best to access the unconscious in his book *The Interpretation of Dreams* (1899). He described dreams as 'the royal road to the unconscious' and as such the best way of gaining access to the unconscious. The idea of 'repression' is central to Freud's conceptualisation of the unconscious. Freud theorised that certain thoughts, feelings and memories are so painful as to be unbearable and are consequently 'repressed' in the unconscious. The process of repression itself is also unconscious.

Freud described his theory on the structure of the mind in his papers 'Beyond the Pleasure Principle' (1920) and 'The Ego and The Id' (1923). Freud proposed that the mind is divided into three separate entities: the id, the ego and the superego. The focus of the id is pleasure, the focus of the ego is external reality and the focus of the superego is morality. Freud postulated that the competing roles of the id, ego and superego lead to conflict which can, if unresolved, lead to psychological manifestations such as depression. Freud also created the concept of 'defence mechanisms' to describe the way in which conflicts between the superego and id can be resolved. For example, denial occurs when someone fails to acknowledge a reality which is unpleasant to them .Other defence mechanisms include reaction formation, projection, intellectualisation and rationalisation.

Freud was controversial in his life-time and his ideas continue to provoke debate over a century after his first published papers. However, his contribution to the development of modern therapy is undoubted given the huge role he played in popularising the value of the 'talking-cure'. Furthermore, although his theories and stages of psychosexual development have been superseded, his legacy in the field of child development is enduring. Freud can ultimately be regarded as the first child development theorist, as it was he who first conceptualised children as passing through specific stages of development. Indeed, Freud's theories formed the starting point of the interest in creating a greater understanding of how children develop. For this reason, it is interesting to be aware of Freud's stages. Freud believed the child had to successfully manage each of these phases before progressing to the next otherwise stagnation occurs at that particular stage and symptoms develop.

Table 16.2 Freud's Stages of Child Development

Oral	0-1	Child's main interest is on oral stimulation
Anal	1-3 yrs	Child's main focus is on defecation
Phallic	3-5 yrs	Child's main focus is on developing sexual identity
Latency	5-12 yrs	Stage of quiescence when there is no specific focus
Puberty	12-20 yrs	The primary focus is relationships with opposite sex

Erikson's Stages Of Development

Erik Erikson (1902-1994) was born in Germany, later moving to Vienna where he became a teacher of art. While in Vienna, he met Freud's daughter Anna, and underwent psychoanalysis. He then decided to train in psychoanalysis. He also trained in the Montessori Method of education, which focused on child development. In 1933, when the Nazis came to power, Erikson emigrated first to Denmark and then to the USA, where he became the first Child Psychoanalyst in Boston. He established a reputation as an outstanding clinician while in Harvard Medical School. He then went to Yale, where he spent time studying and observing children, including a year spent observing on a Sioux reservation in South Dakota, and later while in Berkeley, California, he studied children of the Yurok Native American Tribe.

Erikson is best known for his book *Childhood and Society* (1950). He developed Freud's theory further in a number of useful ways. Erikson's theory was the first to look at development across the life span. He proposed the existence of eight developmental stages in place of Freud's five. Erikson's wife added a 9th stage (old age) before she died, to reflect the increasing life expectancy of western cultures.

Erikson also took greater account of the wider role of society in shaping development, seeing the environment in which a child grew up as crucial to development of identity. Erickson conceptualised development as a series of stages marked by 'crises' - coining the term 'identity crisis' - that had to be resolved to allow the young person successfully cope with the challenges of the next developmental stage.

Erikson won the Pulitzer prize for his book *Gandhi's Truth* (1969) which concentrated on his theory as it applied to later life.

Basic Trust vs. Mistrust (0–1yr)
In this first developmental stage it is essential that the child successfully learns to develop a trusting relationship with others, most importantly parents. If not given this opportunity the child becomes suspicious of others and has difficulty forming relationships.

Autonomy vs. Shame & Doubt (2-3yrs)

In this stage the child needs to successfully cope with the challenges posed by taking more control of behaviour. If the child does not succeed in this the result is a child who lacks self-control and experiences failure.

Initiative vs. Guilt (4–5yrs)
This stage sees the child challenged to develop the drive to self-motivate or alternatively will experience feelings of guilt.

Industry vs. Inferiority (6–11yrs)
The challenge of this stage is for the child to take on different tasks and to learn how to cope with both success and failure. If the child does not learn to accept that failure may occur, it becomes more difficult to cope with any failures and 'failure' may be seen in terms of personal inferiority.

Identity vs. Role Confusion (12–18yrs)
The primary conflict of this stage is for the young person to develop a clear sense of identity in the context of the many different aspects (personal, relational, educational, social and moral) of life. The alternative is a failure to develop a consistent sense of self, leading to role confusion.

Intimacy vs. Isolation (19–25)
The focus of this stage is the challenge posed by forming a close relationship with a partner. The alternative is to avoid taking the chance of a relationship failing and therefore to avoid relationships.

Generativity vs. Stagnation (26–40)
The challenge here is to establish a productive lifestyle, the alternative to which is stagnation.

Ego Integrity vs. Despair (40 years plus)
The challenge posed by this stage is to be able to look back over life with a sense of achievement as opposed to the sense of having wasted life which leads to feelings of despair.

Piaget's Theory Of Cognitive Development

Jean Piaget (1896-1980) was born in Switzerland. He published his first scientific paper at the age of 11 on the albino sparrow. Piaget completed a PhD in Natural Science in Switzerland before moving to France. While there, he taught in a school for boys which was run by Alfred Binet, who had developed the Binet Intelligence Tests. It was while correcting these tests that Piaget formed the basis of his theory. He noticed that younger children consistently got different questions wrong to older children. He hypothesized that younger children were no less intelligent than their older counterparts but rather that they thought differently. He developed his theory through observations of experimental situations primarily with his own children from infancy.

Piaget saw children as 'little philosophers and scientists' constructing their knowledge and understanding. In his view, knowledge was not something that a child simply learned but something that they constructed. This 'constructivist' theory of teaching has had a huge influence in the practice of teaching in both America and Europe leading to a child centred focus. Piaget's view of education was: 'education, for most people, means trying to lead the child to resemble the typical adult of his society…but for me and no one else, education means making creators….You have to make inventors, innovators - not conformists'.

More recent research suggests that Piaget's theories are an underestimate of children's abilities. It is thought that part of the reason for this may be the way in which Piaget derived some of his conclusions. For example, Piaget frequently used experiments with children to assess their thinking. Later research has demonstrated that children in real-life scenarios frequently display more advanced stages of thinking at earlier ages than thought by Piaget.

The stages of Cognitive Development: (Piaget)

The following age-ranges are approximate.

Sensori–motor (0–2yrs)

In this stage the child's experiences are based on motor and sensory stimulation and the child's understanding is based on physical interactions with the world. For example, the child drops a rattle and sees that it falls but does not understand that it is still there. By the end of this stage the child has developed 'object permanence'. This means that the child understands that when an object or person is outside the field of vision or presence it continues to exist and so understands, for example, that when the rattle falls under the table it is still there.

Pre–operational (2–7yrs)

The child's understanding is based on intuitive reasoning. The child starts to use abstract symbols including language to represent objects. Thinking is egocentric and the child cannot see things from another's perspective. At the beginning of this stage, the concept of conservation is absent, however this concept develops during this stage. The child first develops conservation of numbers and then mass. Children in this stage concentrate on only one feature of an object to classify it, dogs have four-legs, therefore all four legged animals are dogs.

Concrete Operations (7–12yrs)

During this stage a child's understanding is logical and concrete. The child is able to classify an object based on more than one attribute. This stage is characterised by thinking which is concrete and based on personal experience.

Formal Operations (12yrs+)

During this stage, thinking transcends the concrete. The child is able to consider multiple dimensions of a condition, allowing consideration and exploration of situations yet to be encountered and make hypothetical assumptions.

Havinghurst's Developmental Tasks (1972)

Havinghurst's theory suggests that there are a number of different challenges or 'tasks' that occur at specific developmental stages. The child must successfully adapt to these challenges to cope with the next stage. The difference in the difficulties that a child may have at various developmental stages is reflective of the different tasks posed by that stage. For example, a young child who is having difficulties coping may be noticed to be slow to learn to walk. A teenager who is struggling to cope may be noticed to have difficulty forming friendships.

Havinghurst's Developmental Tasks

Ages 0–6
* Learning to walk;
* Learning to crawl;
* Learning to take solid food;
* Learning to talk;
* Learning to control the elimination of body wastes;
* Learning sex differences and sexual modesty;
* Getting ready to read;
* Forming concepts and learning language to describe social and physical reality.

Ages 6–12
* Learning physical skills necessary for ordinary games;
* Learning to get along with peers;
* Building wholesome attitudes toward oneself as a growing organism;
* Learning an appropriate masculine or feminine social role;
* Developing concepts necessary for everyday living;
* Developing conscience, morality and a scale of values;
* Achieving personal independence;
* Developing attitudes toward social groups and institutions.

Ages 12–18
* Achieving new and more mature relations with peers of both sexes;
* Achieving a masculine or feminine social role;
* Accepting one's physique and using the body effectively;
* Achieving emotional independence of parents and other adults;
* Preparing for marriage and family life;
* Acquiring a set of values and an ethical system as a guide to behaviour;
* Desiring and achieving socially responsible behaviour.

Moral Development (Kohlberg)

Lawrence Kohlberg (1927-1987) was born in New York. He enlisted in the army in World War II and helped to smuggle Jews to safety in Palestine. When he returned from war, he served as a professor first at the University of Chicago and then at Harvard.

Kohlberg was a follower of Piaget whose work on cognitive and moral development informed his theory. Kohlberg's basic method in categorising the Stages of Moral Development was to give a group of children a number of dilemmas to consider. For example, 'Heinz steals the drug' describes a man called Heinz whose wife was going to die without access to an expensive drug. Heinz could not afford the drug and therefore stole it. Should Heinz have done that?'

Kohlberg was not simply interested in whether the child said 'yes' or 'no' but why and how the conclusion was reached. Based on the answers Kohlberg received, he categorised 3 basic levels of morality, each with 2 subsections.

Level 1: Pre–conventional/Pre–moral

Stage 1: "Avoidance of Punishment"
Kohlberg described this level as 'preconventional' because the child sees morality as external to the self, as a set of rules which he most obey. The child does not speak as a member of society. The child could therefore consider Heinz's response right. 'Heinz can steal it because he asked first and it's not like he stole something big; he won't get punished' or more commonly as wrong. 'It's bad to steal'. When asked to explain why they reached this decision, children in stage 1 of the preconventional level of development, frequently refer to the consequence i.e. the behaviour leads to punishment therefore this makes the behaviour wrong.

Stage 2: "Fairness"
In stage 2 of the preconventional level, children appreciate that there are different points of view, for example, that of the pharmacist and that of Heinz. In this stage, children see punishment not as proof that the behaviour is wrong but as something to try to avoid. Children at this stage typically invoke the concept of 'fairness'. Heinz was right to steal from the pharmacist because 'he was trying to rip him off'. At this stage, the child does not see the moral issues as relating in any way to the wider community and as such is their moral reasoning is labelled as 'preconventional'.

Level 2: **Conventional Morality**

Stage 3: "What others would think"

Children at this stage are usually entering their teens. Young people at this stage are generally concerned that the behaviour and motivation behind it is such that it can be labelled as 'good' and that it is based on positive feelings including love and empathy. For example, 'He was a good man for wanting to save her.' At this stage of moral development, the teenager is cognisant of the views of the wider community: 'Heinz loved his wife and wanted to save her. I think anyone would'.

Stage 4: "Conforming with laws"

At this stage, the young person is concerned with the wider ramifications of the behaviour and its impact on society. Young people at this stage frequently say they understand Heinz's motivation but that his behaviour is wrong because if everyone simply followed their own moral code there would be a breakdown in society. Although respondents in this category frequently see Heinz's behaviour as wrong, similar to in stage 1, the rationale behind their decision is very different. At this stage, the young person appreciates the functions of rules in a society as opposed to simply seeing punishment itself as defining what is right and wrong.

Level 3: **Post–conventional**

Stage 5: "Balance society & self"

At this stage the young person thinks about the essential values that society should try to uphold in reaching a decision. He sees that there are certain basic rights such as the right to liberty and the right to life, which all societies should endorse. Therefore, 'It is the husband's duty to save his wife'. The fact that her life is in danger transcends every other standard you might use to judge this action. Life is more important than property. At this stage, young people are also influenced by the person's duty to society and its laws when injustice should be fixed through a democratic process.

Stage 6: "Individual conscience"

Kohlberg's description of this stage of 'universal principles' reflects that of philosophers such as Kant and leaders such as Gandhi and Martin Luther King. Democratic processes do not always meet the needs of all groups within society. It is very possible for a law to be passed which will benefit some and endanger others. Therefore, the principals of justice must apply to all members of society equally and are therefore universal. To reach this type of moral understanding in practice, Kohlberg suggested that a person simply views the situation through each of the protagonist's eyes as though he did not know which role he would ultimately have to take on. If this happens, it should be possible to reach a just resolution based on universal principles; in this instance the pharmacist would realise that if he had been the person dying, he would not have wanted profit valued above life.

A decade after Kohlberg had developed this theory, he visited a kibbutz and saw the positive influence of kibbutzim on the young people's moral development. As a result, he opened a school, which was run on the principle of a 'just community' where the students had the right to make democratic decisions. He subsequently introduced this model to a number of schools and a prison.

Kohlberg contracted a tropical disease at the age of 44 which resulted in chronic pain and episodes of depression. At the age of 59, Kohlberg took a day's leave from the hospital in which he was being treated and ended his life by suicide.

The influence of Social Context on Children's Development (Bronfenbrenner)

Urie Bronfenbrenner was born in Russia and went to the USA at the age of six. He completed his MA at Harvard followed by his doctorate in the University of Michigan. He then served as a psychologist in World War II. Later he became Professor of Human Development and Family Studies and of Psychology at Cornell University.

Brofenbrenner's 1979 book *The Ecology of Human Development* was ground-breaking in conceptualising child development within an ecological framework. Brofenbrenner proposed that children develop as part of a wider system which encompasses family, culture, society and the world as a whole which is represented by four 'ecological levels'. A child's development must be seen in the context of these wider systems. As children grow they interact with the world around them, shaping environment and in turn being shaped by it. In this way, the child's behaviour is influenced by the wider social environment into which that child is born and grows up.

The microsystem is the setting within which a child is placed at any given time, for example, the home or the creche. As the child grows the number of potential microsystems to which they are exposed increases.

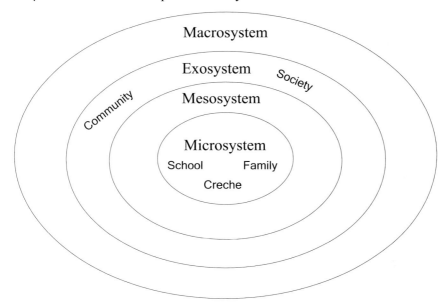

Fig. 16.1   Diagram representing Brofenbrenner's Model

The mesosystem is the interaction between two microsystems within which the child functions, for example the home and the school. The stronger the complementary links between the two the greater the potential impact of that system on the child. For example, if a parent works very closely with a school to facilitate changes in a child's behaviour, the impact on the child is likely to be much greater. Broffenbrenner also emphasises transitions between systems. For example, a child can be facilitated in negotiating changes within a system if they are given advance knowledge as to what the new situation will be, for example, transitions from primary to secondary school.

Hierarchy of Needs (Maslow)

Abraham Maslow (1908-1970) was born in New York, the first of seven children of Russian immigrants. He studied at the University of Wisconsin, where he worked with Harry Harlow. Harlow had carried out very influential work on the attachment behaviours of baby monkeys to their mothers. While observing these monkeys, Maslow noticed a number of specific aspects of their behaviour, which informed his theory. In particular, he was struck by the fact that certain needs take precedence over others. For example, if a monkey is thirsty it will seek to get a drink. However, if it is being choked, as it is experiencing thirst, it will seek to get its breath back first.

Maslow coined the term 'hierarchy of needs' to describe the different levels of need which a child will have. This theory is not developmentally based in that many of the same 'needs' transcend different ages and developmental levels. If basic needs are not met, a child will not be able to reach potential 'self-actualisation'. The first four levels were described by Maslow as deficit or 'd' needs (Biological and Physical Needs, Safety Needs, Belongingness and Love Needs, Esteem Needs). When these needs are not being met, a person will notice the deficit. However, when the need is being addressed the person will not be conscious of that process. In contrast the final stage is described as a 'being need' or 'b' needs (Self-actualisation). These needs motivate the person to pursue their potential and the person is consistently aware of these needs even while pursuing them.

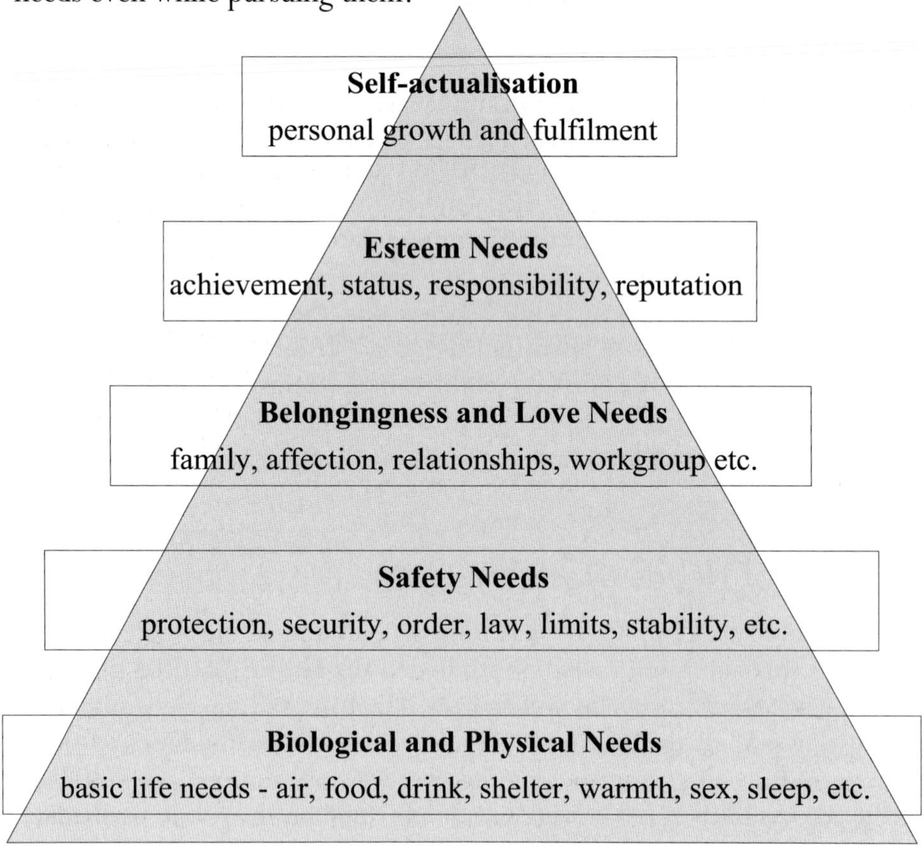

Self-actualisation
personal growth and fulfilment

Esteem Needs
achievement, status, responsibility, reputation

Belongingness and Love Needs
family, affection, relationships, workgroup etc.

Safety Needs
protection, security, order, law, limits, stability, etc.

Biological and Physical Needs
basic life needs - air, food, drink, shelter, warmth, sex, sleep, etc.

Fig. 16.2 Diagram representing Maslow's Model

Theories of Language Development

One of the first recorded papers on the subject was the work of a German biologist Tiedeman (1787) who studied the development of language in children. Almost a century later, Charles Darwin contributed to the field. The work of Preyer (1882) who published a descriptive study of the first 3 years of his son's language development led to a growth of interest in the area, culminating in the huge amount of interest that this subject has generated in the last 20 years.

The 'How' of language development continues to be a hotly debated topic. The different theories can be broadly divided into four groups; the environmentalist and nativist explanations are the two ends of the spectrum. The fullest explanation of language development is most likely to incorporate aspects of all four explanations.

I. Environmentalist explanations

Skinner (1957) proposed a behavioural theory for the development of language. This theory suggests that a child learns to speak through a process of selective reinforcement. In this theory, babbling is crucial to the development of language as it is shaped through repeated reinforcements into approximations of speech, which in turn develops into adult speech, as sounds not consistent with adult speech are not reinforced.

However, behaviourist theory provides an inadequate explanation of language development as it fails to take account of the numerous sounds that a child develops without reinforcement and the child's spontaneous application of grammatical 'rules' in different contexts. e.g. a child will add 'ed' to infer past tense, 'I talked', even when not correct, 'I goed'.

II. Nativist Explanations

This theory was based on the idea that if language development cannot be understood in the context of what is happening 'outside of' the child as proposed by environmentalist theorists, then it could best be understood as coming from 'within' the child. Thus Chomsky (1966) proposed the existence of a Language Acquisition Device (LAD), an area within the brain containing all the universal 'rules' of language systems. This theory proposed that children could learn language with limited amounts of environmental input. This theory has not been supported by subsequent research.

However, ongoing work, taking the 'neo-nativist' approach is continuing to explore ideas that have developed from Chomsky's original theory. Comparative cross-linguistic studies have focused on the idea that there are sets of 'rules' underpinning all languages called 'universal grammar'. It is hypothesised that if the rules of universal grammar were understood, then it would be possible to decipher the developmental process, which occurs in children as they learn language.

III. Cognitive Explanations

Cognitive theorists such as Brown (1973) suggest that while there is much regularity to language development, this does not fully support the conclusion that language development is innate as proposed by nativist theorists. Cognitive theorists link language development to more general learning theory. As the child moves through the Piagetian stages of cognitive development, the complexity of language increases. As the child reaches the formal operations stage, which facilitates hypothetical and abstract thought, linguistic development expands as the young person experiences new ways of using language.

IV. Functional Explanations

Functional theories seek to explain language development in terms of the function it serves in social communication. This theory explains language in the context of a child's desire to communicate. As Halliday (1978) proposes: ' *the individual's language potential is interpreted as the means whereby the various social relationships into which he enters are established, developed and maintained.*'

Table 16.3   Language Milestones

From birth	Crying cooing at 1 month
6-9 months	Babbling
9-12 months	Turn taking, Intonation
1 year	First word spoken, "Holophrase"
18 months	20 words
21 months	200 words
2-3 years	2 word phrases - "telegraphic speech" e.g. "me car"
3-4 years	1000 words
6-8 years	2600 words

Important Concepts In Child Development

Self–Esteem

Self-esteem is extremely important in allowing a child to grow to reach full potential. Self-esteem is defined as the individual's appraisal of self. Self-image and ideal-self are very important components of self-esteem. Self-image is how the young people see themselves and ideal-self reflects the young person's preferred way to be. The young person's self-esteem reflects the difference between the two.

The self-esteem of a child develops in the context of the child's appraisal of life experiences. A child's self-appraisal may include an acknowledgement of poor academic skills but this may be balanced by a positive sense of social competence. Another child might struggle in all domains. A child's self-esteem will also be influenced by the judgement of those close to him or her. For example, one child may struggle with reading but have a parent who ensures that the child is supported appropriately and the child's self-esteem may be unaffected. Another child may be subjected to harsh criticism from parents in the same situation which will have a negative impact on self-esteem.

Myths about Child Development

Nature versus nurture

It is now widely accepted that neither environmental nor genetic factors can provide the sole explanation for the complexity of child development. An interactionist model is widely endorsed. For example, a child who is genetically endowed with a high IQ seeks out stimulation from the social environment from infancy which in turn leads to enhanced cognitive development.

A child's personality can be moulded by parents and environment

There is no doubt that a child can be shaped by environment. However, innate temperament will influence interaction with that environment and how it affects the child.

There is definite 'critical period' in child development from birth to 3 years.

Brain development continues well into early adulthood. To date a 'critical period' has not been scientifically established.

There are no validated developmental screening tools for preschoolers
There are well validated screening tools available to assess young children for developmental delay. These screening tools are very sensitive to detecting developmental difficulties.

Language development: children learn second languages quickly and easily.
The 'critical period' hypothesis has been increasingly questioned in recent years, with many experts suggesting that children's apparent superiority at language acquisition at younger ages may have little to do with biological factors and more to do with social and motivational drives.

Resources

http://cyfernet.ces.ncsu.edu. Children, Youth and Families. Education and Research Network. Practical research based information from the nations leading universities in the USA.

Child Development Institute: Keeping Parents Informed
www.childdevelopmentinfo.com

US Department of Health and Human Services, Centers for Disease Control and Prevention
www.cdc.gov

US department of Education, Office of Educational Research and Improvement: www.ed.gov/offices

Early Childhood information and resources for teachers and parents
www.earlychildhood.com

17 Child Abuse

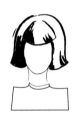

Martha's story

Martha is a 7 year old who has began bed-wetting and is often awakened by nightmares. She is often sexually disinhibited in school with a friend. Her behaviour is aggressive and she becomes distressed for no apparent reason. She is very aware of her surroundings and personal space and becomes angry if anyone accidentally touches her as they pass by...

What is Child Abuse?

Under current Irish legislation a child is defined as someone under 18 years. Child abuse is any act or failure to act that endangers a child's physical or emotional development.

Child abuse can be categorised into four types: physical, sexual, emotional or neglect.

- ➤ Physical abuse is defined as injury to a child resulting from any or all of a variety of acts including hitting, kicking, choking, throwing and whipping;
- ➤ Child sexual abuse may include physical sexual acts or non-contact sexual abuse including exposure to pornography;
- ➤ Emotional abuse is any attitude or behaviour which interferes with a child's mental health or social development. It rarely presents with physical symptoms. It includes prolonged critical comments, sarcasm or hostility and also includes emotional unavailability by the parent to meet the child's emotional needs;
- ➤ Neglect occurs when a child is deprived of food, hygiene, intellectual stimulation, affection and appropriate supervision. Neglect also refers to lack of opportunities for normal healthy development. There are five types of neglect: physical, emotional, medical, mental health and educational neglect.

What signs should the teacher look out for?

- ➤ Watchful, anxious children who are cautious or wary of adults;
- ➤ Inability to play and be spontaneous;
- ➤ Aggression;
- ➤ Underachievement in school;
- ➤ Difficulty trusting other people and making friends;
- ➤ New onset of wetting or soiling;
- ➤ Inability to sleep;
- ➤ Fear of physical contact;
- ➤ Age inappropriate use of sexual talk or ideas in their play;
- ➤ Feeding problems;
- ➤ Over-friendliness with strangers.

What are the effects of Child Abuse?

The effects vary depending on the duration and severity of the abuse and who the perpetrator is. There are more serious long-term effects on the child's development and well-being where the dominant interactions between parent and child have been abusive. In the case of physical abuse, there may be immediate physical effects including haemorrhaging, bruising, suffocation, and broken bones. There may also be long-lasting psychological consequences including a vulnerability to Depression, Anxiety and Eating Disorders. The child may not be able to play imaginatively or interact with peers, have low self-esteem and be self-critical, may not be able to concentrate and make progress in school, and may avoid school activities that involve the removal of clothes. Some children experience Post-Traumatic Stress Disorder (See chapter 10), a combination of symptoms that involves reliving the trauma over and over, avoiding things that remind them of the trauma, anxiety responses and behaviour problems.

What is Munchausen's Syndrome by Proxy?

This occurs when a parent fabricates stories of illness about the child or deliberately causes physical signs of illness. It can occur if the parent secretly administers drugs to the child or inflicts an injury on the child and then invents a story to imply that some underlying and unexplained illness has caused the symptoms.

Physical symptoms which are suggestive of Munchausen's Syndrome by proxy include symptoms which cannot be explained by medical investigation. Munchausen's Syndrome by proxy should also be considered when parents demand medical investigation when there are no apparent physical signs or if urine samples reveal the presence of unprescribed medication or blood.

How serious is the impact of Child Abuse?

Child abuse and neglect may interfere with a child's development in many ways including psychological, academic and physical development. The child's capacity to form and maintain relationships may be negatively affected. It is important to remember that the objective signs of abuse do not always reflect the severity of the abuse, particularly as emotional abuse tends to be cumulative and effects may only be apparent in the longer term. Abused children often suffer low self-esteem, behavioural problems and are at increased risk of juvenile delinquency. They may have interpersonal difficulties and later have difficulty looking after their own children's needs. Some children who are raised in abusive situations may repeat the cycle and be abusive, harsh and punitive. However, other children may grow up and parent in a sensitive and caring way determined to prevent the abuse cycle being repeated. The child's capacity to grow up and break the cycle of abuse is influenced by a myriad of factors including the extent, severity and nature of the abuse and the resilience of the child.

Can any child be abused?

Unfortunately abuse can occur in all socioeconomic groups and at any stage of a child's upbringing. Children are more vulnerable to developing psychological problems if the abuse or neglect is severe, if young when the abuse begins, if they have a close relationship with the abuser, if they blame themselves for the abuse and if they lack social support and coping skills. It is very difficult to establish an accurate figure of the extent of abuse in Ireland but the actual incidence of abuse and neglect is estimated to be three times greater than the number reported to the authorities.

Is child abuse a 'new phenomenon'?

There are numerous descriptions of the abuse of children in literature and references throughout history of the maltreatment of children in its multiple guises. The 'battered child' syndrome was written about in 1860 by Ambroise Tardieu, a French forensic physician.

The *Ryan Report* (2009), graphically illustrates the extent of child abuse in Ireland in the twentieth century and its devastating transgenerational consequences.

What are the risk factors for child abuse?

When assessing risk, it is useful to look at family risk factors and community risk factors. Poverty is the most frequently and persistently noted risk factor for child abuse.

Family Related Risk Factors
- Lack of support for socially isolated families;
- Domestic violence;
- Intergenerational abuse - many children learn violent behaviour from parents and grow up with poor coping skills and end up abusing their own children;
- Personal history of abuse;
- Emotional immaturity;
- Alcohol abuse;
- Drug abuse;
- Unwanted/unplanned pregnancy;
- Poor coping skills;
- Poor problem-solving skills.

Individual Child Risk Factors
- Premature birth;
- Child with intellectual disability;
- Physical impairment;
- Difficult temperament (personality).

Community Risk Factors

Children are at more risk in an area with high unemployment, high rates of crime, poor housing, lack of facilities and drug abuse.

Cultural Factors

Child abuse occurs in all cultures. In some cultures, it is acceptable to physically punish children to discipline them.

Legislation in Ireland

Child Care Act, 1991

This legislation deals with children in need of care and protection. The welfare of children is the paramount principle underlying the act.

UN Convention on the Rights of the Child

Ireland ratified the UN Convention on the Rights of the Child in 1992. The convention is a "bill of rights" for all children. It conveys rights relating to every aspect of children's lives including the right to survival, development, protection and participation. Article 19 of the Convention states that parties shall take all appropriate legislative, administrative, social and educational measures to protect the child from all forms of physical or mental violence, injury or abuse, while in the care of parent(s), legal guardian(s) or any other person who has care of the child.

Guiding Principles from the Children First Guidelines for reporting Child Abuse:

Teachers have a key role in identifying child abuse and neglect and in protecting those at risk. The child must be protected from further abuse in line with Department of Health, Children's First Guidelines.

There are three stages of recognition of child abuse:
- ➤ Considering the possibility;
- ➤ Looking out for signs of abuse;
- ➤ Recording of information.

The safety and well-being of the child or young person must take priority. Reports should be made without delay to a GP or health board. While the basis for concern must be established as comprehensively as possible, children or parents should not be interviewed in detail about the suspected abuse.

If child abuse is suspected, the following steps should be taken.
- ➤ A report should be made to the health board in person, by phone or in writing. Each health board has a social worker on duty for a certain number of hours a day.
- ➤ In the event of an emergency or the non availability of health board staff, the report should be made to An Garda Siochana. This may be done at any Garda station.

Protections for Persons Reporting Child Abuse Act, 1998
This Act includes:

The provision of immunity from civil liability to any person who reports child abuse "reasonably and in good faith" to designated officers of health boards or any member of An Garda Siochana.

The provision of significant protection for employees who report child abuse. This protection covers all employees and all forms of discrimination up to, and including, dismissal.

The creation of a new offence of false reporting of child abuse where a person makes a report of child abuse to the appropriate authorities "knowing that statement to be false". This is a new criminal offence designed to protect innocent persons from malicious reports.

What can the teacher do to help?

Help!

If a child has been abused or neglected, the child needs support in the school environment and consideration needs to be given to the fact that certain emotional difficulties or challenging behaviour the child may display may be related to the abuse suffered.

If a child becomes distressed in class there should be an agreement that a certain safety plan can be activated. For example, the child could go and talk to the home/school liaison teacher or leave the classroom for a few minutes until feeling able to rejoin the class.

Some schools have developed personal safety programmes as part of their Social, Personal and Health Education (SPHE). This programme teaches children how to recognise and avoid abusive situations, where to look for help if in danger and how to develop social skills for developing appropriate relationships with others.

The 'Stay Safe Programme'

The 'Stay Safe Programme' is a personal safety skills programme used in many schools. This was developed in Ireland by the Child Abuse Prevention

Programme which aims to reduce child abuse and bullying through the provision of personal safety education for children, in-service training for teachers and parent education. The programme aims to give children the following:

> ➢ Skills to recognise and resist abuse/victimisation;
> ➢ Knowledge to always tell an adult about any situation in which they feel unsafe or dangerous;
> ➢ Self-esteem and self-protective skills.

It is taught through five different modules using classroom discussion, role-play and repetition. The content of the modules includes feeling safe/unsafe, bullying, touches, secrets and telling and strangers. The overall message is that children should say 'no', get away and always tell an adult.

Safety on the Internet

Children are increasingly using the internet and while it provides a great source of information, there are many dangers if some basic precautions are not taken by parents. Children may accidentally log onto sites with pornographic material, receive unsolicited emails or enter a chat room.

When is professional help needed?

Many abused children will need specialist treatment on an ongoing basis. Many have symptoms of PTSD, Depression, suicidal behaviour and psychological difficulties. Children who experience distress that impairs their ability to carry out everyday school activities and relate to peers and teachers, should be assessed by CAMHS. Children who have been abused are often referred to a specialist child abuse unit for validation that the abuse took place. When the abuse is confirmed, a treatment plan is usually recommended. There are also specialist centres for children who themselves are abusers.

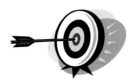

Treatment

Safety skills training is very important for children who have been abused. It is useful to teach coping skills for upsetting thoughts. This usually includes relaxation skills training. The child can be supported to use relaxation skills in multiple situations. It is very important however, that consideration is given to the type of relaxation strategy taught and to ensure that the child feels safe at all times. Some relaxation techniques such as massage may be experienced as threatening by a child who has been abused .

Cognitive Behavioural Therapy
CBT provides explanations for children to understand the experience of abuse; it helps children realise that other children who have been abused experience similar symptoms and difficulties. The therapist teaches the children to label emotions and to understand the relationship between thoughts, feelings and behaviour. The therapeutic work involves cognitive restructuring to help children identify and challenge negative or distorted thoughts that may be the precursors of emotional and behavioural problems. For example, the child may think "It was my fault I was abused, I am no good, I am never any good". The child in this case is encouraged to identify individual strengths while also recognising the extent to which this thought represents a negative, self-critical evaluation which is not based on fact. This process where the child learns to recognise distorted thinking patterns and challenge these beliefs ultimately leads to more balanced thinking. This in turn helps the child accept the statement 'it wasn't my fault'.

Myths

Sexual abuse only happens in lower class or rural families.
Sexual abuse happens across all socio-economic communities and it happens in both city and rural environments.

Children often make up stories or lie about sexual abuse.
While children do make up stories and get confused about specific details, they seldom lie about sexual abuse. Children who have not been abused do not usually have explicit knowledge of intimate sexual behaviour.

The child is to blame for encouraging or allowing the sexual abuse to happen.
Adults are responsible for their own behaviour. A child or young person is never responsible for behaviour displayed by an adult.

Resources

Children at Risk in Ireland, (CARI) Foundation, 110 Lower Drumcondra Road, Dublin 9 Tel: 01-8308529, Fax: 01-8306309, Helpline@cari.ie

Childline Tel:1800 66 66 66

Children First National Guidelines for the protection and welfare of children, department of health and children, September 1999

Child Abuse Prevention Programme (CAPP), The Lodge, Cherry Orchard Hospital, Ballyfermot, Dublin 10, Tel: 01-6206347, Fax: 01-6206347

Commission to Inquire into Child Abuse, Second Floor, St. Stephen's Green House, Earlsfort Terrace, Dublin 2, Tel: 016624444.

Child Protection, Guidelines and Procedures, Department of Education and Science, Primary Circular 0061/2006.

Department of Health and Children, Hawkins House, Hawkins Street, Dublin 2. Tel: 01-6354000, Fax: 01-6354001.

Stay Safe Best Practice in Child Protection. Guidance for Schools. Child Abuse Prevention Programme, Bridge House, Cherry Orchard Hospital, Dublin 10. Email: staysafe@indigo.ie

Support Network for Professionals in Child Protection, c/o 70 Lower Leeson Street, Dublin 2. Tel: 016614911, Fax; 01-6610873

Books

Children First, National Guidelines for the Protection and Welfare of Children, Department of Health, 1999.

Johnson, Charles F. "Abuse and Neglect of Children." In Nelson *Textbook of Pediatrics*, ed. Richard E. Behrman. Philadelphia: W. B. Saunders Co., 1996.

Krugman, Richard D. "Child Abuse & Neglect." In Pediatric Diagnosis & Treatment, ed. William W. Hay Jr. et al. Stamford: Appleton & Lange, 1997.

Leventhal, John M. "Child Maltreatment: Neglect to Abuse." In *Rudolph's Pediatric*, ed. Abraham M. Rudolph, et al. Stamford: Appleton & Lange, 1996.

Social, Personal and Health Education Guidelines. Department of Education and Science, 1999.

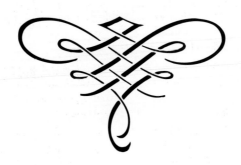

Index

R

referral 13, 45, 56, 69, 78, 110, 120, 157

relapse 109, 111, 136, 138, 140 - 141

relationships 4, 6, 10, 12 - 14, 35, 39, 50, 52 - 53, 57, 59, 66, 82, 93, 104, 108, 111, 129 - 130, 147, 152, 166, 186 - 188, 196, 198, 203

relaxation 45, 120, 129 - 130, 157, 168, 170, 208 - 209

resilience 4, 6, 9 - 10, 19, 144, 204

rules 6, 23, 26, 51, 58, 63 - 65, 67 - 69, 82, 164, 192 - 193, 197 - 198

S

schizophrenia 13, 36, 133 - 142, 176 - 177

self esteem 70, 87, 156

self monitoring 29

sensory 17, 24, 56, 59, 134, 181, 184, 190

separation anxiety disorder 37

serotonin 43, 105, 109, 119, 166, 170, 174, 176

sexual abuse 92, 202, 209

siblings 14, 86

side-effects 29, 105, 139 - 140, 174 - 179

social phobia 36, 42

social skills training 58, 70

socioeconomic 129, 204

special educational needs 7 - 8

specific learning disability 7

sphe 34, 184

St. John's Wort 178 - 179

stigma 4, 6

stress 1, 5 - 6, 9, 34 - 35, 37 - 42, 44, 46, 51, 85 - 86, 89, 100 - 104, 106, 111, 118, 121, 123 - 126, 128, 130 - 132, 136, 138, 141, 144 - 149, 152 - 153, 158, 163 - 164, 168 - 170, 201, 203, 207 - 208

subjective 22, 41, 99, 107

substance abuse 66, 70, 152, 157

suicide 84, 100 - 101, 136, 175, 194

T

temperament 43, 67, 144, 199, 205

therapist 15 - 17, 56, 78 - 79

tic 115 - 122

trauma 9, 102, 119, 124 - 132, 145, 203

treatment 13, 15, 28 - 29, 36, 42, 45 - 47, 67, 70, 84 - 86, 88 - 89, 93, 101, 105, 110, 112, 120, 131 - 132, 134, 136, 138 - 140, 159 - 161, 169 - 170, 173, 175 - 179, 208, 211

triggers 109 - 110, 121, 168

U

underweight 81, 83

V

visual aids 26, 57

vulnerable 56, 85, 87, 102 - 103, 129, 141, 204

W

weight 81 - 83, 85, 87 - 90, 93, 98 - 99, 137, 140, 174 - 176